Essential Microbiology and Hygiene for Food Professionals

Essential Microbiology and Hygiene for Food Professionals

Sibel Roller

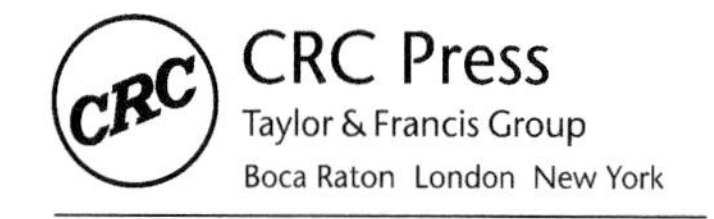

CRC Press is an imprint of the
Taylor & Francis Group, an **informa** business

CRC Press
Taylor & Francis Group
6000 Broken Sound Parkway NW, Suite 300
Boca Raton, FL 33487-2742

ISBN 13: 9781444121490 (pbk)

British Library Cataloguing in Publication Data
A catalogue record for this book is available from the British Library

Library of Congress Cataloging-in-Publication Data
A catalog record for this book is available from the Library of Congress

Visit the Taylor & Francis Web site at
http://www.taylorandfrancis.com

and the CRC Press Web site at
http://www.crcpress.com

Cover image © Elena Schweitzer/Fotolia
Section opener images © DEX Images/Photolibrary Group Ltd/Getty Images (p1), © Richard Cote – Fotolia (p41) and © Lasse Kristensen – Fotolia (p161)

Typeset in 10.5/14 pt Minion by Phoenix Photosetting
Printed and bound in Italy

Contents

Foreword

For too many years chefs have felt that the understanding of food hygiene was either "cissy" or just plain unnecessary. One of the fundamental reasons for this "wrong thinking" has been the boring way that hygiene, and the study of microbiology, has been portrayed in the past. At last we have a book that is easy to read and tells us in a simplified manner what we need to know and to do and does not complicate the issue with excess explanations. We all need to protect those who enjoy the results of our labours in the kitchen. This book tells us how.

Brian Turner CBE

Preface

When I first started teaching food microbiology, I would ask all my new students at the beginning of term if they had received any food hygiene training. A show of hands would tell me that very few had, even among those managing food businesses or working as chefs. Since the turn of the millennium, this has been changing gradually and many food handlers now have, as a bare minimum, some form of basic food hygiene certificate. But a 1-day theoretical course in food hygiene finished off with a multiple-choice test hardly scratches the surface of the vast body of knowledge that exists about controlling foodborne diseases. Of course, a short course is better than nothing but it is not enough to ensure that good hygiene is practised consistently. The fact that it is not is reflected in the millions of preventable cases of food poisoning that occur every year. And contrary to popular belief, food-poisoning symptoms are not trivial. Thousands of people die of foodborne disease every year. Not surprisingly, food-poisoning outbreaks, both big and small, continue to feature prominently in news headlines.

Like other vocational subjects, such as nursing and midwifery, the discipline of culinary arts has risen beyond the craft level to undergraduate and even postgraduate degree levels. Students enrolled on culinary arts courses want to be more than just cooking operatives. They want and need to become knowledgeable about their subject, learn how to critically assess information, become technological innovators and acquire a sense of responsibility for themselves, their customers and the world around them. This book, like the growing discipline of culinary arts, is part of a new drive for excellence in the food profession.

Traditional degree courses in food science, food technology, nutrition and dietetics focus, quite rightly, on the sciences of chemistry, microbiology, engineering and nutrition. These science courses are well served by a range of excellent food microbiology textbooks that delve deeply into microbial physiology and the analytical methods used to detect, identify and manipulate microorganisms in the laboratory. But these books do not meet the needs of students who are interested in food but not necessarily in the minutiae of microbiology. They are too detailed and they often assume substantial prior knowledge of basic science.

This book is different. It is an unashamed introduction to food microbiology at a level that is accessible by students with limited or no science skills. The book provides basic facts about food-poisoning microbes and how to control them without drowning the student in unexplained jargon and impenetrable detail. It is an attempt to stimulate learning while sharing some of the excitement of studying microbiology. It is intended for all those students who need to know about microbiological food safety but are unlikely to ever work in a science laboratory. Students enrolled on food studies courses that include product design, consumer science, public health, marketing, psychology, sensory science, sports nutrition, leisure management, hospitality, event management and so on will find this book useful. The book is also suitable for the newly emerging courses in molecular gastronomy and culinology (a blend of culinary arts and food science). It is aimed primarily at the undergraduate market (foundation and Bachelors' degrees) but it could also be used in Masters' conversion courses.

A note for students

In writing this book, my aim has been to help you, a budding food professional, to learn how to handle food safely and avoid poisoning your clients. To achieve this, you need to know some basic microbiology. This may seem daunting at first, but food microbiology is not difficult if it is explained simply. So don't be afraid, a little help is all you need and, hopefully, it's right here in this book.

Food is about so much more than just survival. It is about pleasure, traditions, culture, fashion, mood, religion, family and friends. But to assure food safety effectively, you need to know a lot of facts. These are so much easier to remember if there is a story to go along with them. When it comes to food poisoning and its consequences, there are plenty of stories to tell. This book tells a few of them. And the personalities who have shaped the history of microbiology also have their stories: these are told in the coloured Halls of Fame textboxes. I hope that you will find the stories enjoyable.

To help with your learning, the book is richly illustrated with photographs, line drawings, cartoons and graphs. The properties of the most important food poisoners are summarized in Microbial CVs and each chapter ends with a selection of tasks, exercises and quiz questions to do on your own or in class. Whenever a new term or technical word is first used in this book, it is printed in **boldface** and explained in the text. Subsequently, if you come across the same term again but have forgotten the meaning, use the glossary at the end of the book to remind you of the definition. A list of abbreviations and symbols is also provided.

Inevitably, some of the information in this book will date rather too quickly. Consequently, you are advised to access the latest information about outbreaks, research, legislation and food policy on the Internet. The web is a veritable treasure-trove of information available anytime, to anyone at the click of a mouse. But beware: the Internet makes no distinction between facts, comments, speculation and plain untruths. There is much misinformation, especially about food, on the Internet. You will need to use your critical skills to distinguish between fact and fiction. To help with this, useful weblinks are provided at the end of each chapter and on the accompanying website.

A note for instructors

Like cooking, microbiology is an intensely practical, hands-on subject. No book, lecture, tutorial or beautifully shot, colour-enhanced image of a microorganism can ever provide the same learning experience as a well-designed practical class in a laboratory. Those 'aha!' moments when students connect theory with practice come much more readily when a course includes a range of practical exercises. These can comprise, for example, light microscopy, isolation of microbes from spoiled foods, culturing, inactivation at different temperatures, assessment of hand-washing techniques, testing of disinfectants and cleaners, swabbing of surfaces, etc. I have been fortunate enough to work in institutions with the laboratory facilities and technical support necessary to provide this kind of deep-learning environment. Sadly, many institutions that teach food-related courses lack such facilities. Nevertheless, it is possible to devise practical exercises based on hand-hygiene routines, cleaning and observation of food-hygiene behaviours without access to a laboratory. I would urge all instructors to use this book in conjunction with a set of practical exercises, however simple.

This book is not intended to serve as a comprehensive reference source. The number of references, particularly to the primary scientific literature, has been kept to a minimum to avoid distraction from the main messages. However, some suggestions for further reading are given at the end of each chapter.

I hope that you will find this book useful in your teaching and I would welcome comments or suggestions for improvement from colleagues.

Sibel Roller
Microbiologist

(Not a small biologist but a person interested in very small, preferably invisible, living things)

Acknowledgements

A book such as this is impossible to produce by one person alone. I owe a big 'thank you' to all my colleagues at the University of West London and London South Bank University for their advice, encouragement and support. I am particularly indebted to Professor David Foskett MBE, Head of the London School of Hospitality and Tourism at the University of West London, for his vision and recognition of the importance of food microbiology in the culinary arts curriculum.

I wish to thank the book reviewers, who provided constructive criticism of the initial idea for the book as well as the drafts of the chapters. Their suggestions have greatly improved the final product. I am grateful to all the talented scientists and artists who have given permission to reprint many of the images used in this book.

My thanks go to Naomi Wilkinson, Commissioning Editor, and Mischa Barrett, Project Editor, at Hodder Arnold for their patience, even after the umpteenth request for a deadline extension. I would like to thank all my students, past and present, undergraduate and postgraduate, for enriching my life with their diversity and making my job as an educator so rewarding. And last but not least, I thank my husband Marek and son Max for tolerating, with good humour, my endless disappearances to work on 'The Book'. To them, I dedicate this book.

Sibel Roller

How to access the website

This book has a companion website available at

www.hodderplus.co.uk/essentialmicrobiology

To access this content, which includes PowerPoint slides, interactive MCQs, a comprehensive image library and essential web links, please register on the website using the following access details:

Serial number: vwhuf1

Once you have registered, you will not need the serial number but can log in using the username and password you will create during registration.

Section I: Appetizers

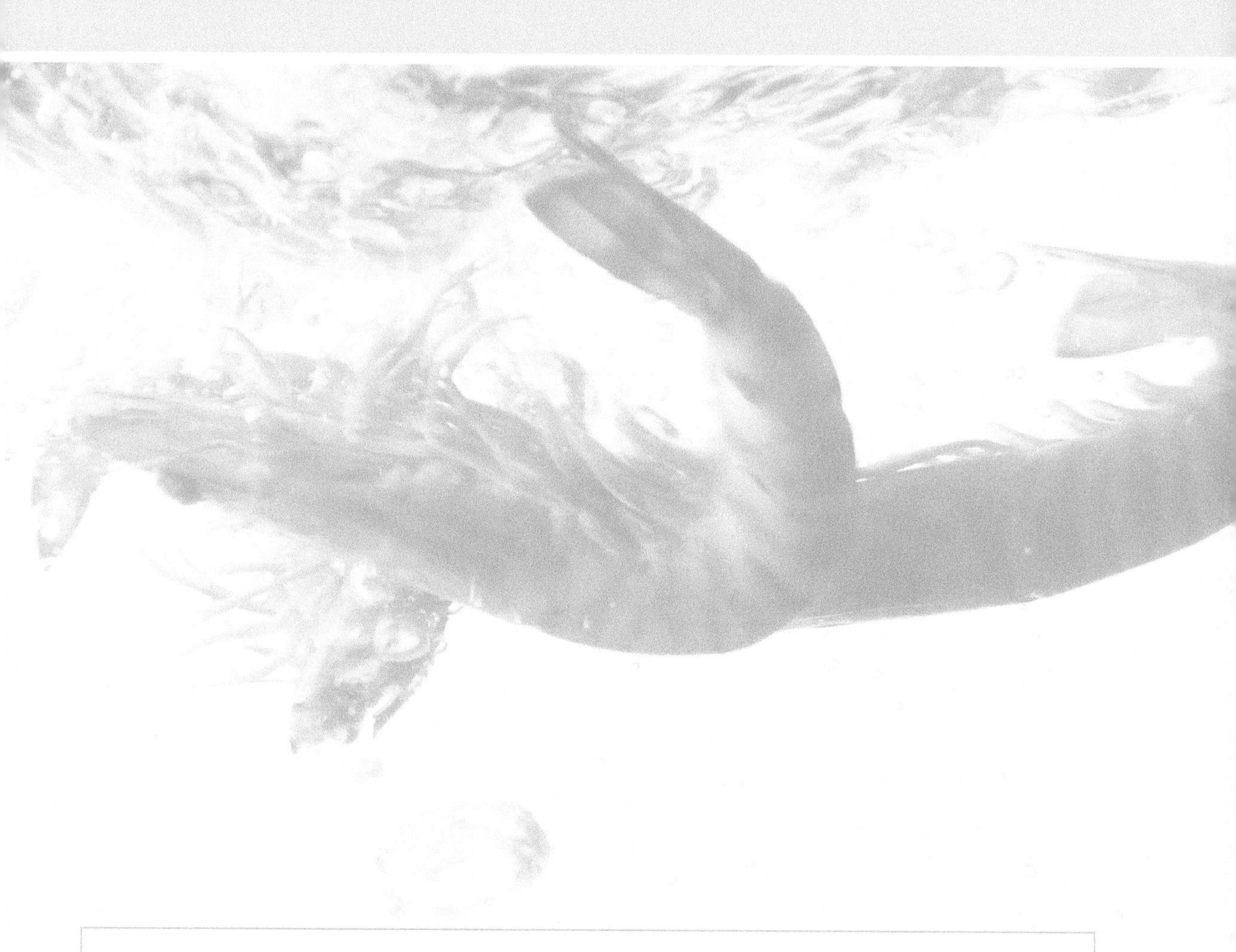

'Hurry, hurry to the parade

Of the strangest creatures ever made.

No legs, no fins, no mouths, no eyes,

Little beasties of the tiniest size.'

Arthur Kornberg,
Nobel Prize winner, 2008

Introduction: The good, the bad and the ugly of the microbial world

Microorganisms (or microbes for short) are all around us but they are so small that they cannot be seen by the naked eye. We need a microscope to see them, so it is not surprising that their presence often goes unnoticed. Microbes are in the air we breathe (Fig. 1.1), the water we drink and the food we eat. The human body is home to millions of microbes that have adapted to live on our skin, nails and hair as well as inside our nose, mouth and gut.

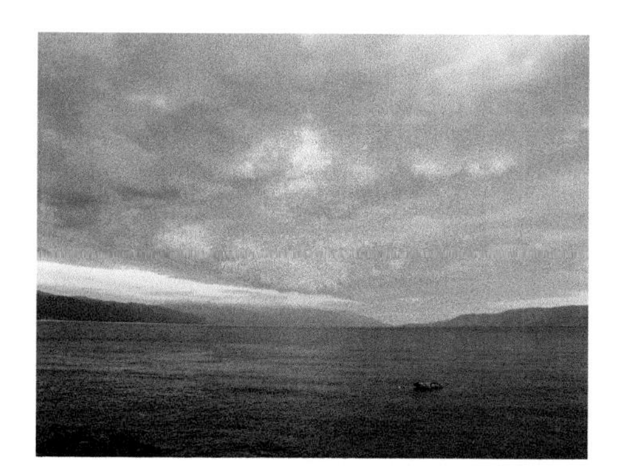

Figure 1.1 Some bacteria can propel themselves around the world in clouds by clinging to water droplets and dust particles.

Some microbes are very hardy and can survive extreme temperatures ranging from hot volcanic pools to near-freezing pockets of brine beneath thick layers of ice. The deepest ocean trenches support a rich microbial life despite high pressures, high levels of salt and toxic minerals, and a complete absence of oxygen and sunlight. Some heat-loving microbes can't grow at all below 85°C, preferring a cosier habitat of at least 110°C or above! At the other extreme, Antarctic explorers have found rich soups of bacteria growing in pools of brine beneath 65 metres of ice. One of the toughest bacteria on Earth, *Deinococcus radiodurans*, can survive radiation doses thousands of times higher than those that kill humans.

In the last few decades, astronomers have discovered more than 500 new planets and several of these may be suitable for life. If we ever find life on some of these planets, it is much more likely to be microbial than in the form of little green men. In 1996, bacteria-like shapes were discovered inside a Martian meteorite that crash-landed on Earth in prehistoric times. This led some scientists to speculate that there may have been microbial life on Mars several billion years ago. Others have disputed this theory and have argued that the Martian 'fossils' were just orderly arrangements of mineralized rock formed during the meteorite's journey to Earth. Whatever the true origins of the life-like forms, there is no theoretical reason why a bacterial spore, buried beneath the surface to shield it from deadly cosmic rays, could not survive the red planet's average temperatures of -60°C for many years. In the further reaches of our solar system, the deep ocean hidden beneath the ice on Jupiter's moon Europa and the subterranean caverns full of water on some of Saturn's moons could also, in theory, support microbial life.

But before we get completely lost in space, let's get back down to Earth! Microbes were the first life forms on Earth many millions of years ago and will probably still be here long after we are gone. In the words of Bernard Dixon 'Microbes, not macrobes, rule the world'.

The good, the bad and the ugly food microbes

Most microbes are harmless to humans and many of them change food in a useful way. We use microbes in the form of starter cultures to turn milk into yogurt and cheese, meat into chorizo sausages and salami, and vegetables into gherkins and sauerkraut (Fig. 1.2). Many beverages and condiments, such as beer, wine, vinegar and soy sauce, would not exist without the action of 'good' microbes.

Some microbes cause illnesses in animals, plants and, most importantly, humans. In terms of numbers, these microbes are in the minority but because of their powerful impact on human health and survival, their study and control

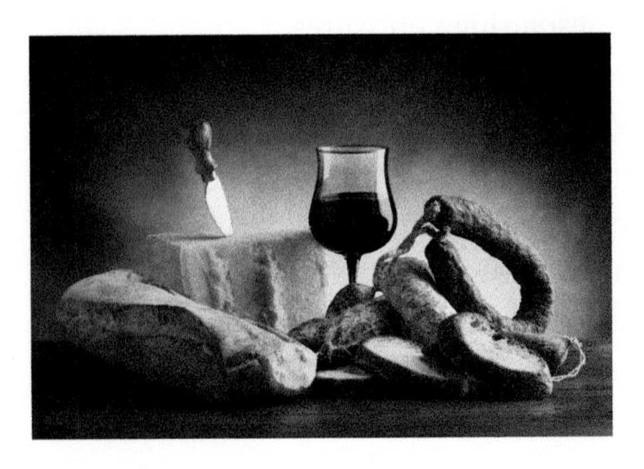

Figure 1.2 Bread, cheese and wine would not exist without the 'good' bacteria, yeasts and moulds in starter cultures (© Marco Mayer, Fotolia).

attracts our attention. These invisible enemies may be tiny but they are capable of killing organisms many times their size and weight. This is reflected in the amount of space devoted to disease-causing organisms in this book.

Between one quarter and one half of the world's food supply is lost after harvest due to bacterial and fungal attack. While microbial spoilage of food may not kill or make anyone ill, it costs industry and consumers many millions of pounds/dollars/euros annually and represents a huge waste of the planet's resources. This is the 'ugly' side of microbial life. As with food poisoning, prevention is better than cure, so the control chapter in this book (Chapter 8) applies equally to food spoilage as well as food-poisoning microbes.

How safe is our food?

Historically, chemical adulteration of food for fraudulent purposes was common. The bread, tea and beer of Dickensian London bore little resemblance to the products we know by these names today. In the late nineteenth and twentieth centuries, new laws were introduced in many countries rendering food adulteration illegal and punishable through the criminal process. These laws have greatly reduced the extent of deliberate food adulteration, although it still happens occasionally. For example, in 2010, unscrupulous traders in China added melamine to milk, leading to the deaths of several babies and young children. However, in terms of sheer numbers of people affected, microbial contamination of food presents a much greater risk than either deliberate or accidental contamination by chemicals.

When it comes to food safety, there is no room for complacency. False confidence and a lack of attention to detail are far more widespread than criminal activity.

There are many myths and misconceptions surrounding the safety of our food. Three examples are given in Box 1.1.

Food poisoning is bad for business

Whether or not people are made ill from eating a food company's products, a food recall can be devastating for business and can lead to bankruptcy and closure. Here are three examples of catastrophic food-poisoning outbreaks and their consequences on the businesses concerned:

- More than a million chocolate bars were recalled by Cadbury's in the UK when *Salmonella* was discovered in 2006 in the chocolate crumb used to make them. The outbreak infected 42 people, including babies and young children. The recall is estimated to have cost Cadbury's £15 million (US$22.5 million).

Box 1.1 Myths and misconceptions

True or false?
'A lot of unnecessary fuss is made over food poisoning. If you get a bit of a stomach-ache, you should just pull yourself together and get on with your life. It's not exactly serious, like cancer or heart disease.'

False
The World Health Organization (WHO) estimates that foodborne and waterborne diseases kill about 2. 2 million people annually, 1.9 million of them children. And it's not just a problem of the developing world. In the UK, more than 1.3 million cases of food poisoning are reported to health authorities each year (and the real number of cases is much higher as many bouts of food poisoning are not reported). Over 20 000 of these cases are hospitalized and nearly 500 people die. About 48 million Americans (1 in 6) get sick every year and, of these, 128 000 end up in hospital and 3000 die from foodborne diseases. These figures are unacceptably high because food poisoning is preventable.

True or false?
'Large food companies are taken to court and may get fined millions of pounds/dollars/euros for making people ill. But most food businesses are small. They can't be punished as they simply don't have the money to pay the fines!'

False
Owners/managers of small food businesses may not be able to pay high fines but they can be sent to jail for making people ill. For example, a kebab house owner in Bradford, England, was jailed for a year after 324 of his customers became ill and 60 were taken to hospital with food poisoning by *Salmonella* originating in his restaurant's chicken doner kebabs. Fortunately, no one died. In addition to the jail sentence, the owner was banned from being a manager, director or employee of a food business for life. His restaurant was closed and he had to pay the costs of the investigation that led to his arrest and prosecution.

True or false?
'A little bit of dirt is good for you, as it helps your immune system from developing allergies, so there is no need to be scrupulously clean in the kitchen.'

continued ➢

False

This view is sometimes referred to as the 'hygiene hypothesis'. In 1989, Dr David Strachan, a London-based epidemiologist, reported that allergies such as hayfever and childhood eczema were more common in small families than in those with large numbers of children. Strachan went on to speculate that infection in early childhood through unhygienic contact with brothers and sisters protected children in large families from developing allergies in later life. He took his explanation one step further by suggesting that improvements in household and personal cleanliness also reduced opportunities for infection and so may have contributed to the increase in allergic diseases seen in many industrialized countries in the twentieth century.

In the two decades following the publication of Strachan's paper, many researchers have attempted to prove or disprove his hypothesis but the scientific evidence has been contradictory and inconclusive. We are still no closer to understanding the reasons why some allergic diseases are increasing in many developed countries. While the increase is real, there are many possible explanations other than the 'hygiene hypothesis'. Meanwhile, the uncritical acceptance of the 'hygiene hypothesis' has led to the popular but overly simplistic notion that we have become 'too clean for our own good'. At a time when food-poisoning incidents preventable by good hygienic practices are unacceptably high worldwide, the 'hygiene hypothesis' should not be used as an excuse for poor hygiene standards.

Another £20 million (US$30 million) were required to undertake safety modifications in the production plant. The company was also fined £1 million (US$1.5 million) and ordered to pay £152 000 (US$228 000) in legal costs after a case was successfully brought against it by Birmingham City Council. Chocolate sales dropped by 14 per cent following the outbreak. The source of contamination was eventually traced to a leaking pipe in the production plant that would have cost just £140 (US$210) to repair.

- The 2006 Dole baby spinach outbreak of *Escherichia coli*, traced to Californian produce, led to five deaths. A further 200 people were hospitalized across the USA. The outbreak cost the spinach industry US$350 million (£230 million) and a lot of disgruntled customers. Two years after the outbreak, spinach sales were still down by 20 per cent.
- In 2008, *Listeria* in cooked deli meat from the Canadian company Maple Leaf Foods left 22 people dead and another 35 in hospital. The company initiated a voluntary recall before the contamination was traced to its own premises but was nevertheless forced to pay 27 million Canadian dollars (US$ 25.5 million; £17 million) in damages.

Major outbreaks such as the examples above attract much publicity but are the large food manufacturers mainly responsible for the highest numbers of food-poisoning cases? Or is it the fault of the retailers with their vast and complex international distribution systems? Or are home cooks mainly to blame? Or could it be that the responsibility lies with the catering profession? Figure 1.3 suggests that in at least one country in the developed world, more than 80 per cent of food-poisoning outbreaks can be traced to caterers working in restaurants, hotels and institutions such as nursing homes, schools and nurseries.

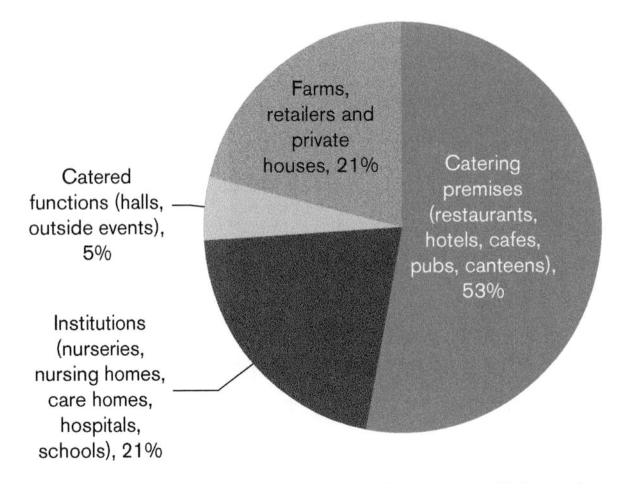

Figure 1.3 Main sources of food-poisoning outbreaks in the UK. Data from UK Health Protection Agency (HPA).

Most deadly car crashes are not caused by badly designed roads, potholes or speed cameras but by people driving carelessly. Similarly, food-safety lapses are rarely caused by faulty cooking equipment, hot kitchens or excessive paperwork but by people preparing food carelessly.

Absolute food safety is impossible to guarantee. But it is possible to *control* microbes sufficiently to minimize risk provided we get to know them! Learning about microbes and their properties is what this book is all about. Safe food-handling practices, informed by knowledge, can help reduce the burden of foodborne disease.

People don't help to keep food safe

People spread germs

Chapter 1 Exercise

The differences between home cooking, catering and food manufacturing

Complete the boxes in this table to the best of your ability. Discuss your answers with a colleague or another student in your class. Then check your answers against the completed table in the Appendix of this book.

Differences in:	Home cooking	Catering	Food manufacturing
Scale			
Timing			
Location			
Accountability when things go wrong			
Possible consequences			

Further reading

Dixon, B (1994). *Power unseen: How microbes rule the world.* WH Freeman, Oxford.

Stanwell-Smith, R and Bloomfield, S (2004). *The hygiene hypothesis and implications for home hygiene.* International Scientific Forum on Home Hygiene/NextHealth, Milan.

This extensive review is over 200 pages long, includes over 500 references and is available from: **http://www. ifh-homehygiene. org/**

Weblinks

For the World Health Organization (WHO) food safety pages, visit:
http://www. who. int/foodsafety/en/

For the latest statistics on food poisoning in the UK and USA, visit:
http://www. hpa. org. uk (UK Health Protection Agency)
http://www. cdc. gov (US Centers for Disease Control and Prevention)

2

Life unseen: The anatomy of microbes

Size matters

Microorganisms, or microbes for short, are living creatures so small that most of them are invisible to the human eye. In order to see microbes, we need a microscope, which magnifies their images to make them look larger.

All animals and plants are made up of **cells** like a house is made up of bricks. Cells are the building blocks of life. Humans have at least 200 different types of cell inside them. Some specialized cells work together in large numbers to form organs such as the liver or tissues such as muscles. Like microbes, animal and plant cells are too small to be seen by the naked eye. They must be magnified at least 100 times (100X) in order to see them.

Microbes such as **bacteria** and **yeasts** are smaller than animal and plant cells. The magnification needed to see bacteria is at least 400X and often 1000X. Grouping microbes according to shape and size is the essential first step in identifying them.

A typical plant or human cell is about 20 μm wide (1 μm is one millionth of a metre). Sperm cells are much smaller, at around 5–6 μm, while the human egg is bigger at around 120 μm. Bacteria are often less than one tenth of the size of an average animal cell. Viruses are several thousand times smaller than bacteria. The different sizes of human cells, plants and microbes are compared in Fig. 2.1.

You could fit around 130 human red blood cells, 200 baker's yeast cells, 1000 bacteria or 100 million viruses inside the dot on top of this letter 'i'.

Humans are home to many bacteria, which live on our skin and in our digestive system. The bacteria in our gut are thought to weigh about 1 kg and outnumber our own cells by 10 to 1. In fact, one could argue that our bodies are more bacterial than human!

The light microscope

A light microscope is the standard piece of equipment used in laboratories to observe microbes and other cells. There are several types of light microscopes but the most common one is the **bright field microscope**, which forms a dark image

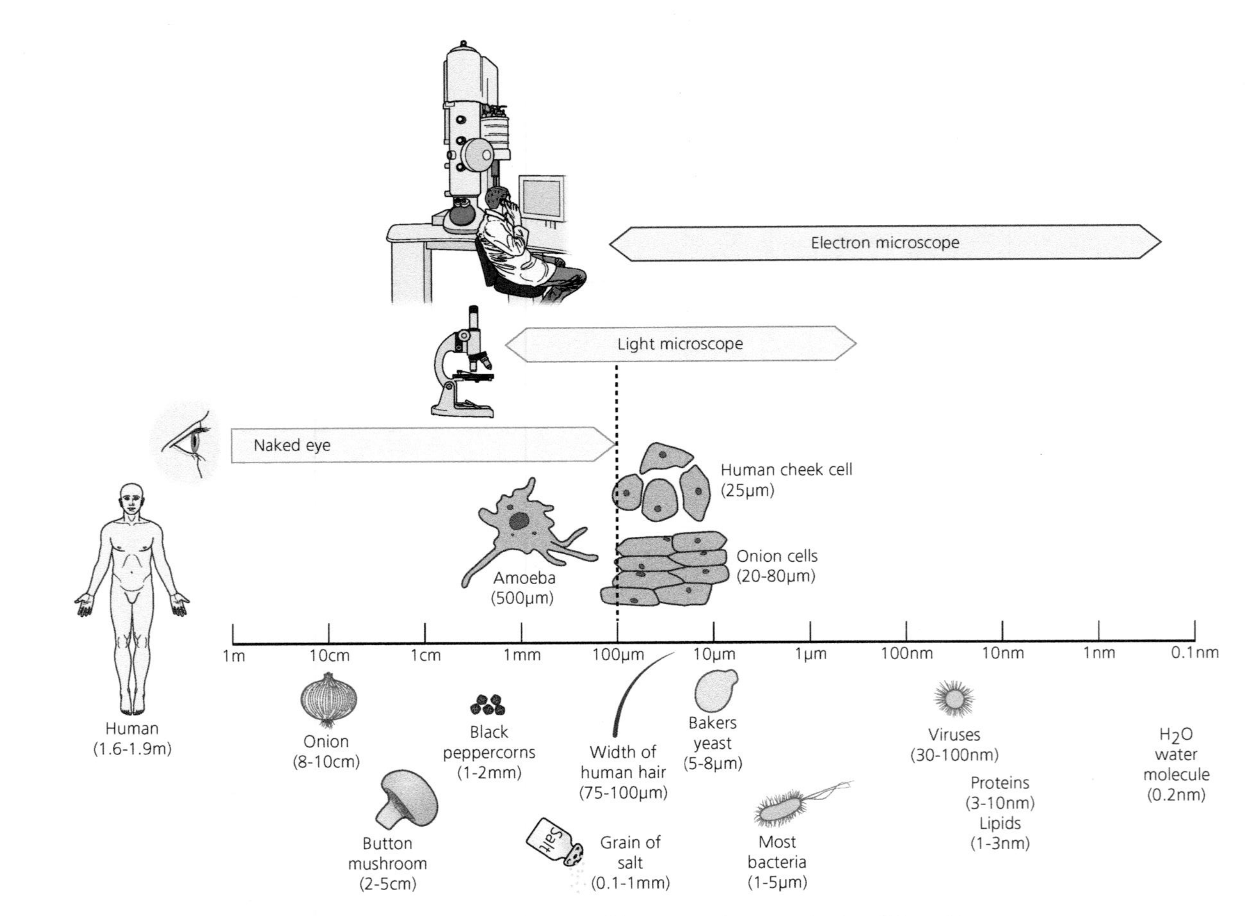

Figure 2.1 Size matters. Comparison of microbial cell sizes with those of humans, plants and other living things. 1 metre (m) = 1000 millimetres (mm) = 1 000 000 micrometres (μm) = 1 000 000 000 nanometres (nm).

against a lighter or brighter background. All modern light microscopes are known as compound microscopes because, unlike their historic predecessors, they enlarge images using more than one magnifying lens.

A specimen or biological sample needs to be mounted on a glass slide for examination under the microscope. The specimen may be from the nose, throat or wound of a sick patient or it may be from a food suspected of causing illness. Saliva, **sputum** (mucus coughed up from lungs), blood, urine, faeces and samples from tissues can all be examined under the light microscope. Microbes grown in the laboratory are usually mounted on glass slides in the form of a 'smear'. Several drops of water with microbes suspended within them are smeared on to a glass slide, allowed to dry and then fixed to the slide by heating the slide in the flame of a Bunsen burner. Figure 2.2 shows the materials needed to prepare slides for microscopy.

A typical light microscope is shown in Fig. 2.3. The light source is located at the base of the microscope. The specimen slide is placed on the stage of the microscope. The condenser, located between the light source and the stage, focuses a cone of light on to the glass slide. Coarse and fine focusing knobs on the side of the microscope allow the adjustment of stage height to produce a clear image. The specimen is viewed through the eyepiece and one of the three magnification lenses. The total magnification of an image is calculated by multiplying the objective magnification by the lens magnification. For example, if a 40X objective is used with a 10X eyepiece, the overall magnification of the specimen is $40 \times 10 = 400$. The maximum magnification achievable by most routine light microscopes is 1000X.

Many microbes are difficult to see even with the help of a microscope because they are colourless and almost transparent. The standard light microscope simply does not provide enough contrast to see cells easily, even for those of us with perfect 20/20 vision! So, microbiologists use several dyes to stain (colour) cells and

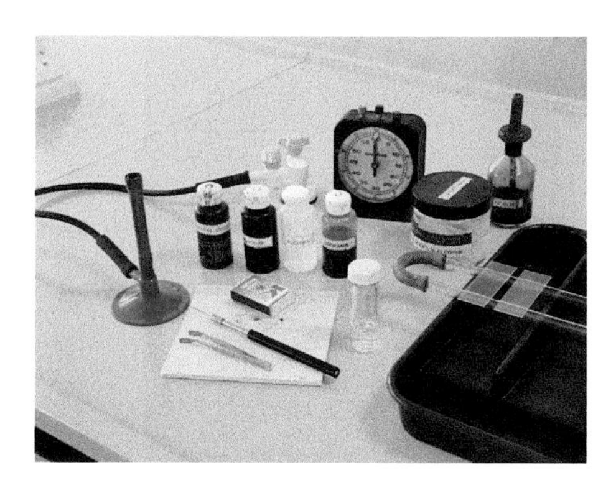

Figure 2.2 Preparing slides for microscopy. A typical laboratory workstation includes (from left to right): Bunsen burner for sterilizing tools; tweezers for handling glass slides; metal loop for transferring bacteria to glass slide and matches on heat-resistant mat; staining materials (crystal violet, iodine, alcohol, saffranine and water); stop-clock; jar containing glass slides; methylene blue; glass slides on staining rack.

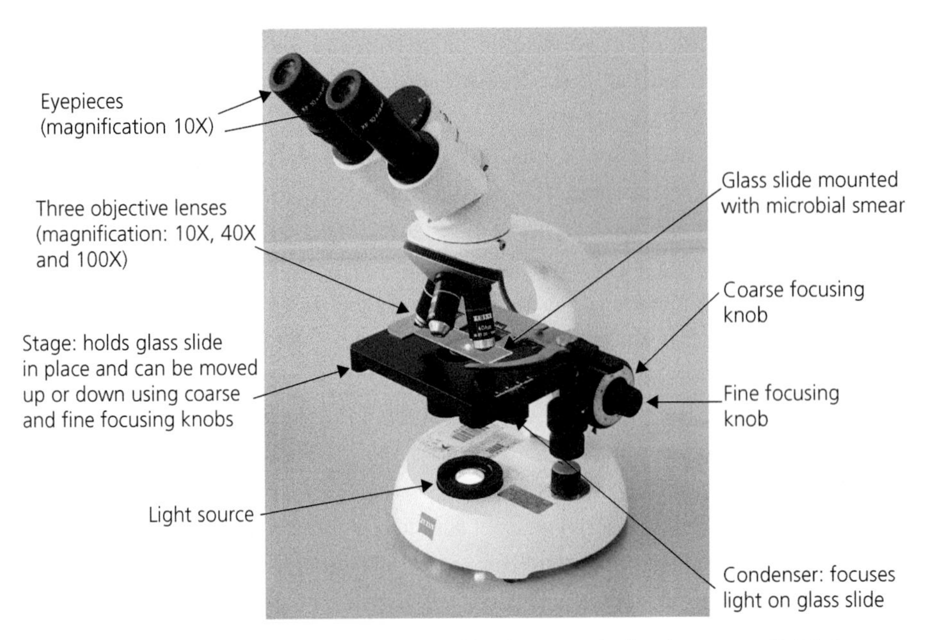

Figure 2.3 A typical light microscope magnifies images of microbes up to 1000 times (1000X).

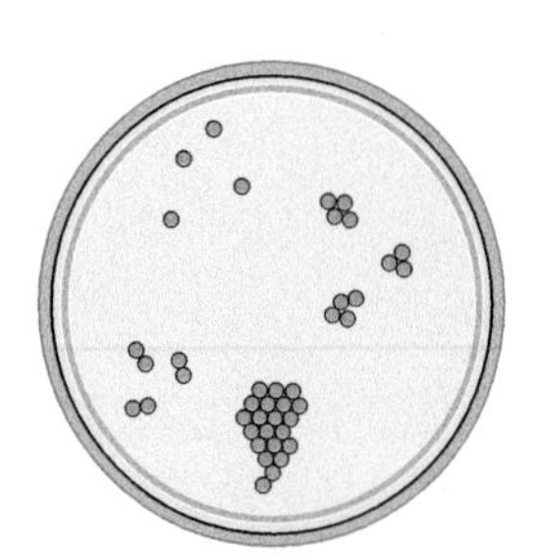

Spherical bacteria: the cocci

Cells occur individually, in pairs, in groups of four (tetrads), or in grape-like bunches

Example: *Staphylococcus aureus*

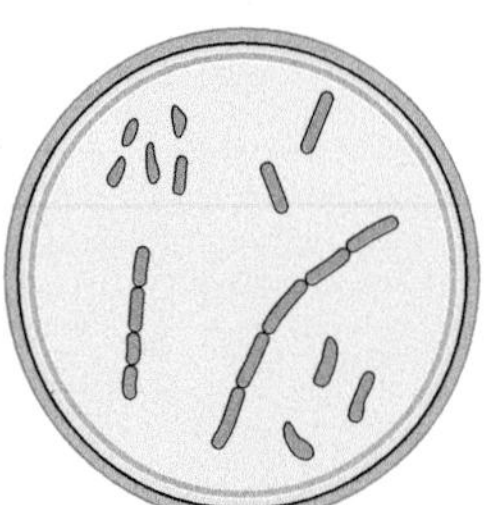

Rod-shaped bacteria: the bacilli

Short or long rods occur individually or in chains

Example: *Salmonella* spp.

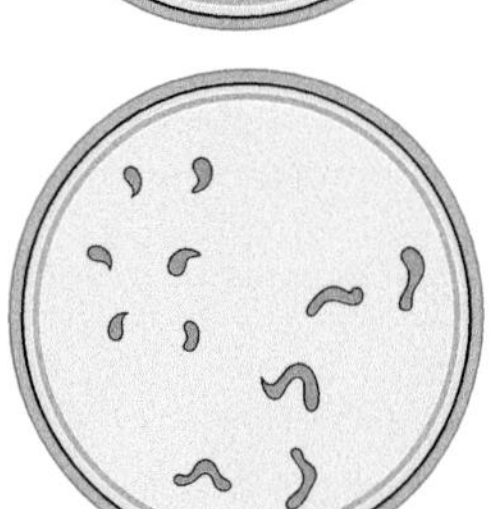

Curved or helical bacteria

Cells are comma shaped or curved (spirillar)

Examples: *Vibrio cholerae* and *Campylobacter jejuni*

Figure 2.4 Bacterial shapes as seen under a light microscope.

improve contrast in microscopic images. For example, simple stains such as methylene blue can be used to colour cheek cells blue, while iodine solution can be used to stain onion cells yellow.

Light microscopy makes it possible to distinguish between different types of cells and microbes on the basis of size and shape. Many bacteria come in two basic shapes: spheres or cocci (singular **coccus**) and rods or bacilli (singular **bacillus**). These are often grouped together in pairs, chains and clusters, as shown in Fig. 2.4. For example, staphylococci are spherical and often appear as microscopic bunches of grapes, while salmonellae are short rods. Some bacteria take on the shape of a comma (*Vibrio*) and others are long rods that have been twisted like a corkscrew (*Spirillum*).

The Gram stain in light microscopy

Gram staining is named after Christian Gram who developed the procedure in the nineteenth century (see Box 2.1). The technique serves two purposes. First, the dyes

Box 2.1 Microbiology Hall of Fame: **Christian Gram (1853–1938)**

Hans Christian Joachim Gram was a Danish physician widely credited with the development of the differential method of staining bacteria now known as the Gram stain.

While working in a hospital in Berlin in 1884, Gram investigated different ways of visualizing bacteria from the lungs of patients who had pneumonia. This serious and often deadly illness is caused by a variety of different microbes, each one requiring different drug treatments. So, in order to select the appropriate medicine for each patient, it was important to identify the causative organism correctly.

Several methods of staining cells to make them easier to see under the microscope already existed. For example, Robert Koch (see Box 3.1) had developed methods for staining the bacilli responsible for causing the often deadly tuberculosis. But visualizing bacteria in samples of sputum, the 'pus' produced in the lungs of infected patients, was difficult because the human cells present in sputum would also react with the stains.

When Christian Gram developed his staining technique, the detailed structures of bacterial surfaces, or indeed the contents of their interiors, were not known. These were discovered in the twentieth century as increasingly sophisticated scientific techniques and instruments revealed the inner workings of cells. The differences between Gram-positive and Gram-negative bacteria are now understood on a molecular level.

Gram's early work was on red blood cells and he was also interested in pharmacology, medical education and the history of medicine. He received many prizes and honours during his illustrious career.

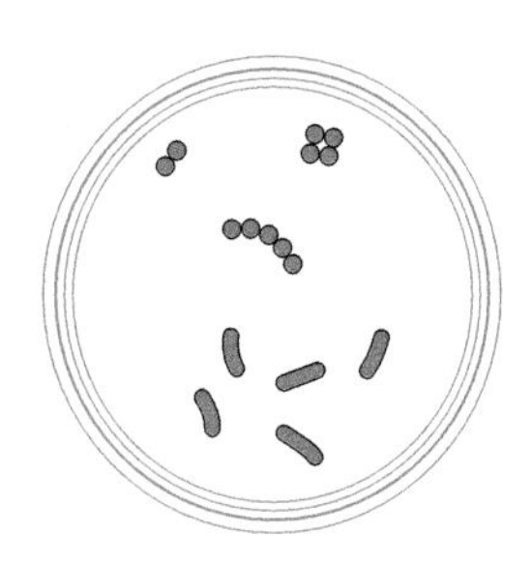

Step 1. Stain with crystal violet

Prepare a smear of bacteria on a glass slide. Heat-fix using Bunsen burner. Flood with crystal violet dye for 2 minutes.

ALL CELLS PURPLE

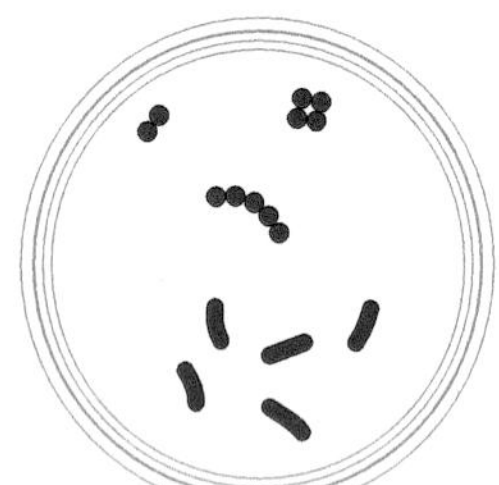

Step 2. Fix with iodine

Pour crystal violet away and add iodine solution for 1 minute. Purple colour intensifies.

ALL CELLS REMAIN PURPLE

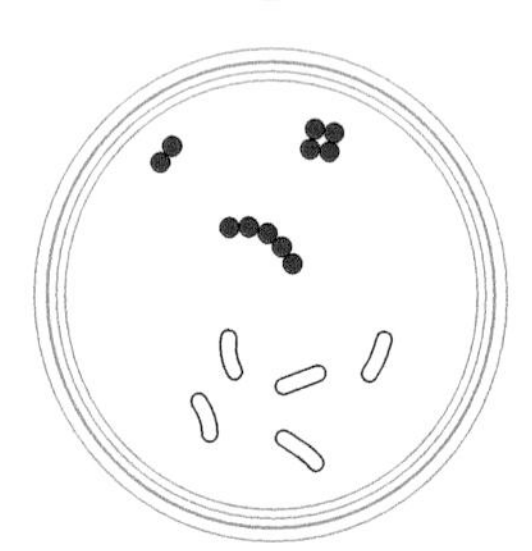

Step 3. Decolourize with alcohol

Wash off all dyes with alcohol and rinse with water.

GRAM-POSITIVE BACTERIA REMAIN PURPLE

GRAM-NEGATIVE BACTERIA BECOME COLOURLESS

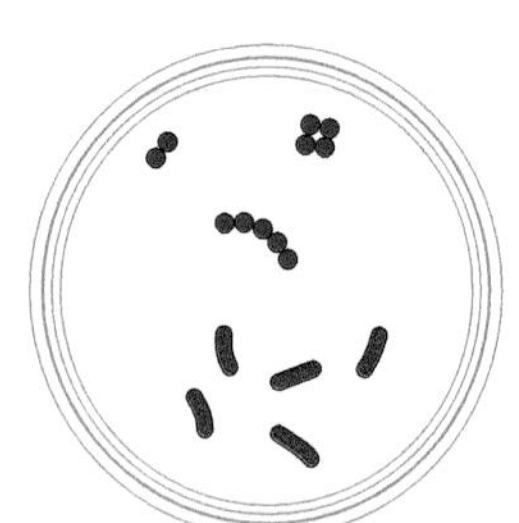

Step 4. Counter-stain with saffranine

Add saffranine dye for 2 minutes. Rinse with water.

GRAM-POSITIVE BACTERIA REMAIN PURPLE

GRAM-NEGATIVE BACTERIA STAIN PINK

Figure 2.5 The four basic steps of Gram staining.

provide contrast and so help us to find the bacteria in the viewfinder of the microscope more easily. Second, the two dyes, crystal violet and saffranine, colour bacteria differently (hence they are known as **differential dyes**). This makes it possible to classify bacteria into two distinct groups that differ in the composition and structure of their **cell walls**: Gram-positive or Gram-negative organisms. Knowing whether a bacterium is Gram positive or Gram negative is the first step in identifying an unknown organism from the environment, the human body or food.

Gram-positive bacteria are purple and Gram-negative bacteria are pink following staining with Gram dyes. A summary of the Gram-staining procedure is shown in Fig. 2.5 and a typical laboratory work station used during staining is

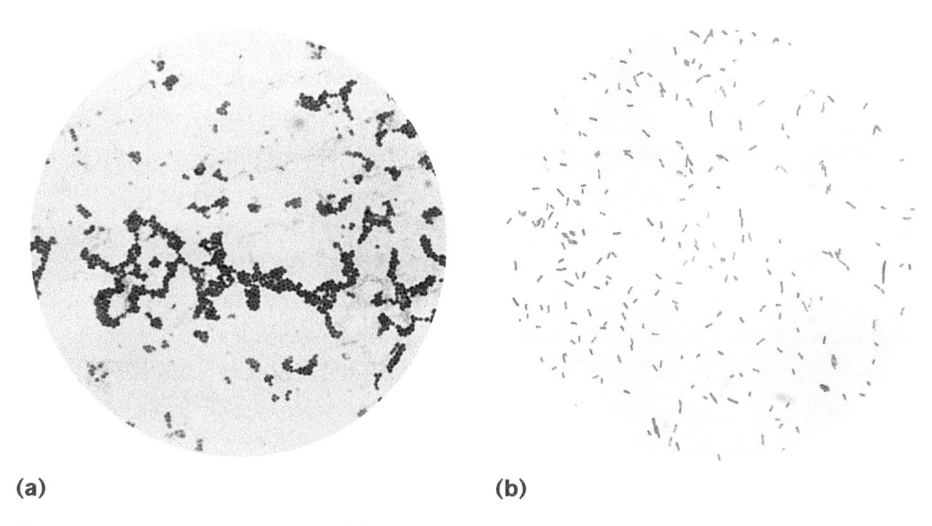

Figure 2.6 Gram-positive cocci (a) and Gram-negative rods (b) magnified 250 times under the light microscope. Figures courtesy of Centers for Disease Control and Prevention (CDC)/Dr Richard Facklam and Larry Stauffer, Oregon State Public Health Laboratory, Oregon, USA.

shown in Fig. 2.2. Images of Gram-positive cocci and Gram-negative rods as they would appear under a microscope are shown in Fig. 2.6.

Bacterial surfaces are extraordinarily complex and play a very important role in the ability of bacteria to cause disease and survive in the environment.

Both Gram-positive and Gram-negative bacteria have fairly rigid cell walls. The cell walls give bacteria their different shapes and protect them from mechanical damage and environmental stresses.

The cell walls of Gram-positive bacteria are made up of thick layers of **peptidoglycan**, a three-dimensional polymer resembling a stack of fishing nets. Each layer is made up of chains of alternating units of **amino sugars** cross-linked with another layer by a short chain of peptides. Peptidoglycan comprises about 90 per cent of the cell wall in Gram-positive bacteria. Gram-negative bacteria also have layers of peptidoglycan but these are much thinner, amounting to just 10 per cent of the cell wall. The Gram-negative layers have fewer cross-links and so are weaker than those in Gram-positive bacteria. The thick peptidoglycan layers of Gram-positive bacteria retain the crystal violet–iodine complex during the decolourization step with alcohol (Step 3, Fig. 2.4), while the more leaky Gram-negative peptidoglycan releases it readily, to be washed away by water.

Bacterial spores

Some Gram-positive bacteria form **spores**. These structures are internal to the cell and so are known as **endospores**. They are faintly visible under the light microscope as unstained spore-shaped regions inside Gram-stained cells. The outer coating of spores is tough and quite stain resistant, so specimens need to be heated in the presence of specialist stains such as malachite in order to colour the spore coat green. A schematic diagram of spores and their position within bacterial cells is shown in Fig. 2.7.

Bacterial spores are very hardy and resistant to heat, dehydration, chemical disinfectants and many forms of radiation, including sunlight and X-rays. Bacteria produce endospores when environmental conditions make it difficult for the 'mother cells' or **vegetative cells** that produced them to survive. Like the seeds of a plant, endospores lie dormant until the conditions are right for them to germinate and produce new vegetative cells. Some spores are known to have survived in the environment for several thousands of years.

Bacterial spores are very important in food microbiology because several spore-forming bacteria such as *Clostridium botulinum* and *Bacillus cereus* are capable of causing food poisoning. Indeed, *C. botulinum* produces one of the most powerful natural **toxins** (poisons) known to man. The properties of foodborne spore formers are covered in more detail in Chapter 7.

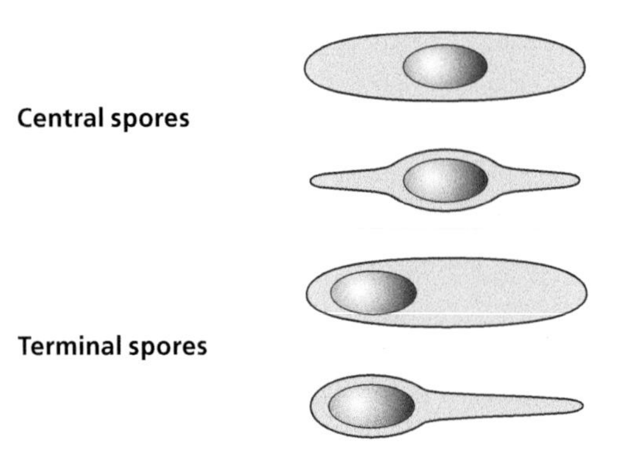

Figure 2.7 Bacterial spores and their positioning within bacterial cells. Examples of spore-forming bacteria: *Clostridium botulinum* and *Bacillus cereus*.

Fungi (yeasts and moulds)

Yeasts and moulds are **fungi**, a group of organisms that is very different from the bacteria in terms of structure. Indeed, the fungi are more like plant and animal cells than bacteria. Like animal and plant cells, the genetic material in fungi is contained within a nucleus surrounded by a membrane. In addition to the nucleus, the fungi have many other internal structures called organelles (similar to organs in a human). Organisms with these complex internal structures are known as **eukaryotes** while the relatively simple bacteria are known as **prokaryotes**. The differences between eukaryotes and prokaryotes are illustrated in Figs 2.8 and 2.9.

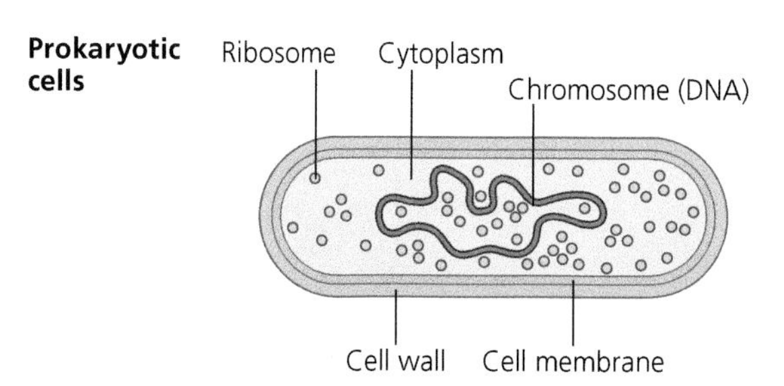

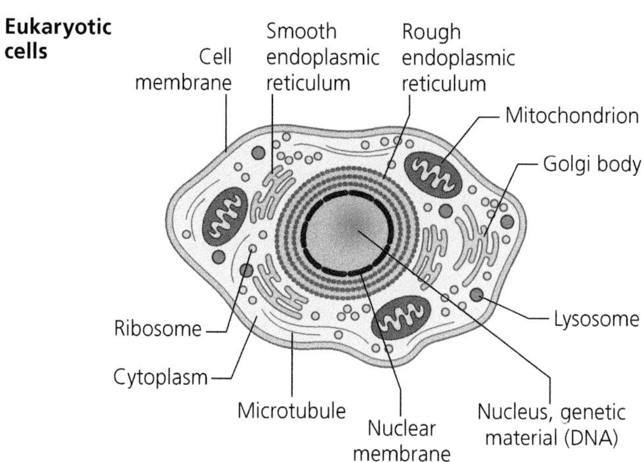

Figure 2.8 The internal structures of prokaryotic (bacterial) and eukaryotic (plant, animal and fungal) cells. DNA, deoxyribosnucleic acid; RNA, ribonucleic acid.

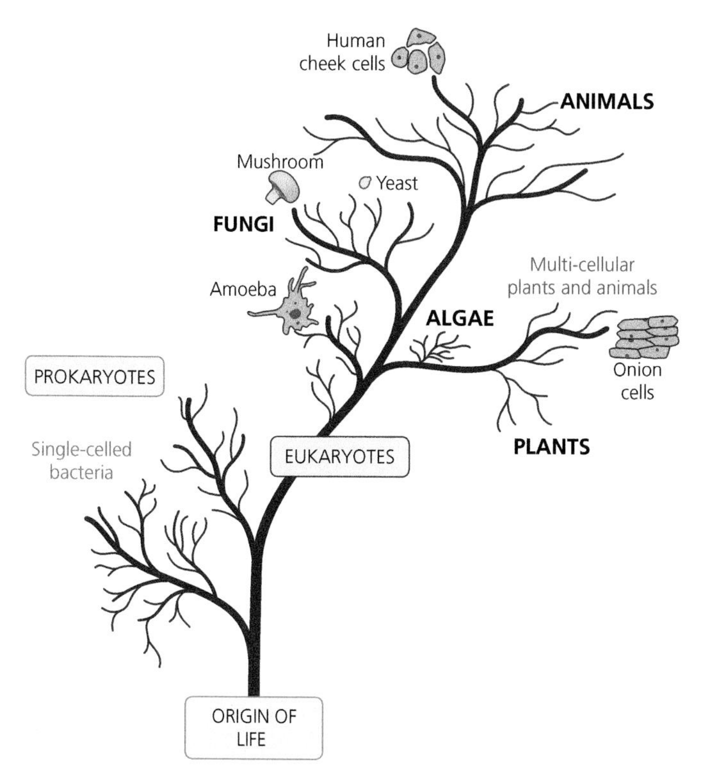

Figure 2.9 The tree of life or the relationship between microbial, plant and animal cells. Note the absence of viruses, which have no cells, from this diagram.

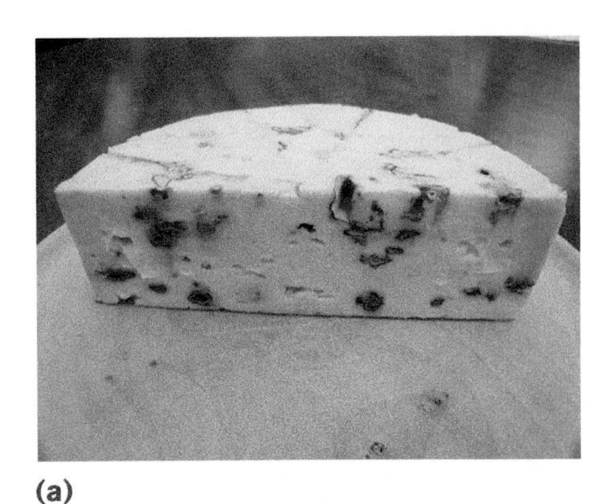

(a)

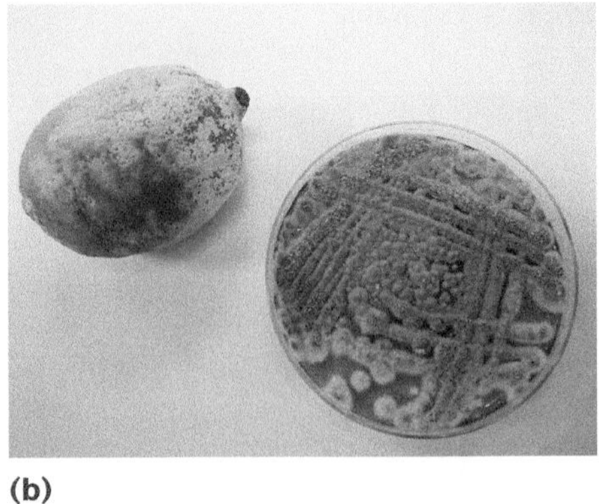

(b)

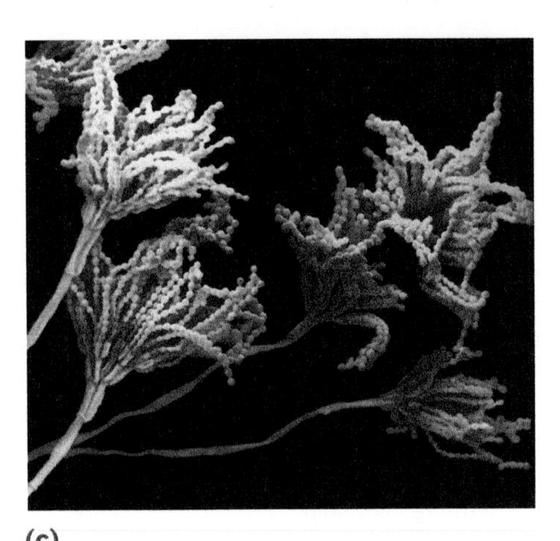

(c)

Figure 2.10 The different faces of *Penicillium* mould. (a) Blue-veined cheese made with *Penicillium roquefortii*. The blue lines on top of the cheese show where the cheesemaker has injected the starter culture. (b) A mouldy lemon spoiled by *Penicillium chrysogenum* and the same fungus grown on agar in a laboratory Petri dish. (c) *Penicillium roquefortii* as seen under an electron microscope. The long branch-like structures (hyphae) have cross walls (septae) and produce bead-like chains of spores (conidia). Magnification: 825X. (© Dr Fred Hossler/Visuals Unlimited, Getty Images.)

The fungi can be divided into two groups: the single-celled ovoid yeasts and those producing filaments or **hyphae (moulds)**. Hyphae are branched, thread-like tubular structures about 10–50 μm in diameter. While yeasts cannot be seen without the help of a microscope, the hyphae of moulds form a fluffy mass of cotton wool-like growth called **mycelium**. These woolly fungal colonies are often visible on mouldy fruit, vegetables or bread. Some examples of fungal mycelia can be seen in Figs 2.10 and 2.11.

Like the spore-forming bacteria, many fungi produce both vegetative cells and spores. Fungal spores are known as **conidia** and are often coloured as in the black spores of *Aspergillus* mould (Fig. 2.11). Unlike the bacteria, many fungi produce

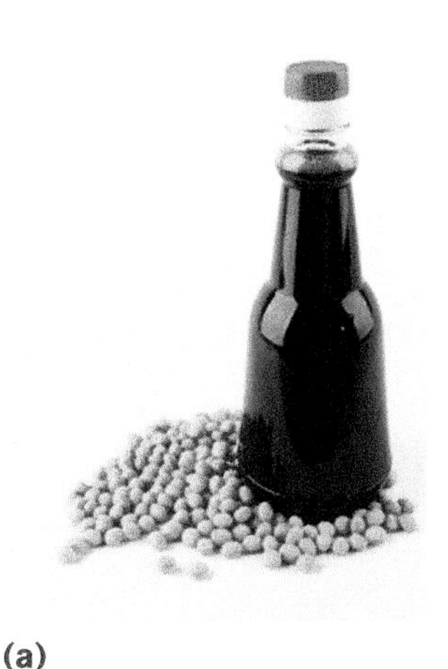

(a)

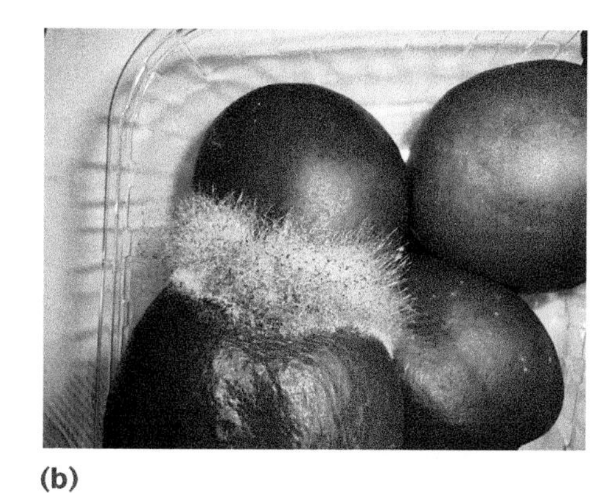

(b)

Figure 2.11 The different faces of *Aspergillus* mould. (a) *Aspergillus sojae* and *Aspergillus oryzae* are used as starter cultures to make soy sauce from soya beans (© chungking, Fotolia). (b) Nectarines spoiled by *Aspergillus niger*. The mass of thread-like white filaments (hyphae) has black fruiting bodies (conidiophores) at the ends of the filaments. These are tiny but visible to the naked eye. The fruiting bodies contain hundreds of spores (conidia). (c) *Aspergillus* as seen under the electron microscope. The single fruiting body (conidiophore) seen in this image bursts open to release hundreds of spores (conidia) into the surrounding air. Magnification: 8000X. (© Dr David M Phillips/Visuals Unlimited/Getty Images.)

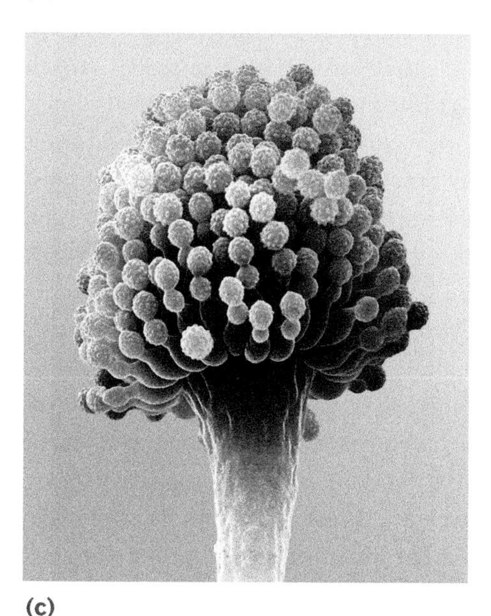

(c)

hundreds of spores within specialized structures known as fruiting bodies or **conidiophores**. The common field mushroom is a fruiting body of the fungus *Agaricus bisporus*. Oyster mushrooms, shiitake, boletus and chanterelles are macroscopic examples of edible fungal fruiting bodies. Examples of microscopic fruiting bodies of *Penicillium* and *Aspergillus* are shown in Figs 2.10 and 2.11.

Beyond the light microscope: microbial structures under the electron microscope

Light microscopy makes it possible to distinguish between yeasts, moulds and bacteria on the basis of size and shape. It also makes it possible to distinguish between different groups of bacteria with the same shape by differential staining such as Gram staining. The routine laboratory microscope is relatively cheap to buy and maintain and the techniques used to prepare samples for microscopy are quick and easy to perform by a trained microbiologist. However, light microscopy has limited capacity to show the fine structure of microbes.

Light microscopy has limited ability to distinguish between objects that are close together. This is referred to as **resolving power** or **resolution**. The resolution limit of the human eye is about 0.2 mm. This means that objects smaller than 0.2 mm cannot be seen and any two objects closer together than 0.2 mm are not seen as separate objects. The best resolution achievable using a light microscope is 0.2 μm. Since most bacteria are no bigger than 1–2 μm, and many are much smaller than this, only their general shape and major features can be seen using the light microscope. The fine internal structures of bacteria cannot be seen under a light microscope. Some microbes such as viruses cannot be seen at all using the light microscope (Fig. 2.1).

In order to see the fine structure of microbes, an **electron microscope** is required. This sophisticated tool can magnify objects up to 100 000 times and can resolve objects that are as close together as 1 nm. The first electron microscope was developed in 1933 by Ernst Ruska. His work was recognized in 1986 when he was awarded the Nobel Prize for Physics. Instead of using glass lenses to bend and focus light rays, electron microscopy relies on magnetic lenses to focus an electron beam on a specimen and so produce enlarged images of very small objects. In modern electron microscopes, the electron beam is fired from an electron 'gun' and focused by doughnut-shaped magnets on the specimen, mounted on a tiny copper metal grid. Since electrons can be deflected by air molecules, air is pumped out of the microscope chamber to create a vacuum. Once the electrons have passed through the specimen, they are captured on a screen or on photographic film to give a magnified black and white image. As most biological materials would be destroyed by this kind of treatment, lengthy and complex procedures have been developed to prepare specimens for electron microscopy.

There are two types of electron microscopes. The transmission electron microscope allows the study of internal structures of microbes while the scanning electron microscope is used for observing the surfaces of microbes. Transmission electron micrographs of *Listeria monocytogenes* and *Clostridium botulinum* are shown in their Microbial CVs in Chapters 6 and 7. A scanning electron micrograph of *Escherichia coli* is shown in its Microbial CV in Chapter 6.

Electron microscopy has enabled scientists to visualize many of the internal structures shown in Fig. 2.8. We now know that all bacteria have:

- A **cell wall** lined with a cell membrane and filled with **cytoplasm**. The composition of the cell wall has been described in the section on Gram staining above.

- A **cell membrane**, also known as a plasma membrane. This is a thin, flexible envelope that separates the cell interior from the external environment. The membrane is just 7 nm thick and consists of lipids and proteins. It is semi-permeable to allow transport of nutrients into the cytoplasm as well as the export of waste materials out of the cell. Water moves in and out of the cell through pores in the membrane. The cell membrane detects and responds to changes in the environment. It also allows cells to communicate with each other.
- A jelly-like **cytoplasm** fills the cell interior and contains proteins, lipids, carbohydrates and inorganic molecules suspended in water.
- A **genome**. Like all living things, microbes contain genes, the hereditary material that contains all the information necessary for the cell to survive and reproduce. In bacteria, several thousand genes made up of tightly coiled strands of **deoxyribonucleic acid (DNA)** are strung together like beads in a necklace to form a single chromosome. The DNA, like a detailed recipe for a cake, contains all the instructions needed for life.
- **Ribosomes**. These important molecular machines are involved in making **proteins** using **ribonucleic acid (RNA)** as messenger molecules to translate the language of the genes into proteins.

In addition to the above structures, some bacteria also have:

- **Flagella**. These long, whip-like tails rotate and help the bacteria to 'swim' or move in liquids. Examples of flagella on *Campylobacter* and *Salmonella* are shown on their Microbial CVs in Chapter 5.
- Hair-like **pili** or fringe-like **fimbriae**. These tubular protrusions are thinner and shorter than flagella and help the bacteria to stick to inanimate surfaces and attach to human and animal cells in the gut.
- **Capsules**. These gel-like coats protect some bacteria from dehydration, chemical attack or the immune system when they find themselves inside an animal or human. They also help bacteria to stick to all manner of surfaces, both inert and alive.
- **Plasmids**. In addition to the main chromosome, some bacteria also have small, ring-like genetic structures known as plasmids; these can shuttle genes between organisms and are one way of spreading antibiotic resistance.

Yeasts and moulds also have many of the structures associated with bacteria, such as cell walls, cytoplasm and membranes, all of which can be visualized using the electron microscope. However, the internal structures of fungi are far more complex than those found in bacteria. In addition, the fungi have specialized organelles not seen in bacteria (Fig. 2.8). Most notable of these is the discrete nucleus, the gene-containing organelle that, at 5 μm in diameter, is considerably bigger than many bacteria.

The structure and life cycle of **viruses** are very different from those of bacteria, yeasts and moulds. Viruses are the smallest of all the microbes and range in size from 20 to 300 nm. They cannot be seen with the light microscope. Viral structures can only be studied using electron microscopy. Compared with bacteria, viruses have a simple structure. This usually consists of a protein coat wrapped around the genetic core made up of DNA or RNA. An example of an electron micrograph of a virus is shown in Fig. 7.2. But don't be fooled by their simple structure: some viruses can be deadly! Their growth and infectious properties are described in more detail in Chapter 7.

Without electron microscopy, viruses and the fine structures of bacteria would be unknown to us. However, electron microscopes are about one hundred times more expensive than light microscopes and require highly skilled personnel to prepare the specimens and operate the equipment. The electron microscope remains the preserve of large research-intensive universities and highly specialized research institutes or analytical laboratories.

Newer forms of microscopy are continually being developed and have improved our ability to observe microbes and their structures. For example, phase-contrast and fluorescence microscopes are now common in routine microbiological laboratories. The atomic force microscope, a more recent innovation, uses a sharp probe and laser beams to visualize surfaces down to the molecular level. Examples of atomic force micrographs of *Salmonella* and *Campylobacter* are shown in their Microbial CVs in Chapter 5.

Protozoa and algae

The majority of **protozoa** and **algae** live in fresh water or seawater and are harmless in terms of human health. However, some species are foodborne and a few have been responsible for food-poisoning outbreaks.

Protozoal infections by species of *Cryptosporidium*, *Cyclospora* and *Giardia* are common in tropical climates but relatively rare in temperate zones except when introduced on imported foods (see Chapter 7). The protozoa are single-celled eukaryotic organisms that produce spherical cysts from 4 to 12 μm in diameter. These resistant cysts can be identified by microscopic inspection of faecal samples from affected patients.

The microscopic algae, like their macroscopic relatives, make energy from sunlight by the process of photosynthesis. The microscopic **dinoflagellates** produce toxins (poisons) that can accumulate in shellfish such as oysters and mussels during periods of 'algal bloom' or 'red tide'. The poisons do not harm the shellfish but can lead to paralytic shellfish poisoning in humans who eat them.

What's in a name?

With thousands of different types of plants, animals and microbes all around us, it is necessary to have a system of naming and organizing them into groups. Some scientists, known as taxonomists, devote their whole careers to naming, grouping (or classifying) and identifying organisms. This is important not just for academic purposes. The correct identification of species is essential in order to trace the spread and locate the source of infection during a food-poisoning outbreak. Further details about identifying microbes correctly are given in Chapter 4.

The Swedish physician and naturalist Linnaeus was one of the earliest taxonomists and he introduced the binomial system of naming living things way back in the eighteenth century. Using this system, animals, plants and microbes are given scientific names consisting of two parts. The first part is the genus name and the second part is the species name. Like a human family with the same surname and many individual members each with a first name, a large genus can have many individual species within it.

The full scientific name for humans is *Homo sapiens*; *Homo* is the genus and *sapiens* is the species. Unlike the genus *Homo*, which has just one surviving species (*sapiens*), many microbial genera are groups of several, and sometimes numerous, related species. An example of this is the genus *Listeria*, which includes five species but only one of them, *Listeria monocytogenes*, is responsible for food poisoning.

Some species can be further subdivided into very closely related but different strains. For example, baker's and brewer's yeast are different strains of the same species *Saccharomyces cerevisiae*.

Microbial names often have Greek or Latin roots describing their appearance or their preferred habitat. Some are named in honour of the scientists who discovered them. For example, *Escherichia coli* was named after Theodor Escherich, a paediatrician working in Graz and Vienna in the early part of the twentieth century. He devoted himself to the study of intestinal diseases in children (*coli* means from the colon, or gut). Similarly, *Salmonella* is named after the American veterinarian Daniel Salmon who developed a vaccine against a pig disease caused by this microbe.

Binomial names are always printed in italics with the genus name starting with a capital letter. In handwritten documents, such as laboratory workbooks, the names are underlined. Since scientific names can be rather long (and sometimes difficult to pronounce!), they are often abbreviated (e.g. *E. coli)*. When reference is made to several or even all the species in a genus, the abbreviation 'spp.' is often used after the genus name (e.g. *Salmonella* spp.). When a freshly isolated microbe has not been identified to species level but its genus is known, the abbreviation 'sp.' is used (e.g. *Salmonella* sp.). Note that the abbreviations 'sp.' (singular) and 'spp.' (plural) are not italicized.

Like most of science, microbial taxonomy is not static and so microbial names change occasionally. The need to rename organisms may arise when new data become available about the properties or genetic make-up of particular strains. For example, in the 1980s, it was recognized that the 2000 or so species of *Salmonella* reported in the scientific literature were in fact so similar that they could be combined into just two species: *Salmonella bongori* and *Salmonella enterica*. The latter was divided into six subspecies, of which the food-poisoning *Salmonella enterica* subsp. *enterica* is the most important in terms of human infections. The previously named species were then renamed by their serotype (an identification method based on antibodies, see Chapter 3) culminating in mouthfuls like *Salmonella enterica* subspecies *enterica* serovar Enteritidis. Such long, cumbersome names are abbreviated by using the genus initial in italics followed by the capitalized serotype without italics (e.g. *S.* Enteritidis). This new system of naming *Salmonella* spp. makes perfect sense to microbiologists but tends to confuse students and members of the public alike! Consequently, the generic name *Salmonella* is used throughout this book except when the complete species and strain name are absolutely necessary to avoid confusion.

Chapter 2 Quiz

Testing your knowledge

1. What different types of microbes are there? Name as many groups as you can think of.
2. What are the differences between bacteria, yeasts and moulds? (Tip: Comment on the differences in shape, size and internal structures.)
3. Can you use a standard light microscope to see 'flu' viruses? Explain your answer.
4. Why is it important to know whether bacteria are Gram negative or Gram positive?
5. Are microbial cells visible under a standard light microscope?

Further reading

There are several excellent food microbiology textbooks on the market intended primarily for university students with some basic knowledge of chemistry and biology:

Adams, MR and Moss, MO (2007) *Food microbiology*, 3rd edn. Royal Society of Chemistry, Cambridge.

McLauchlin, J and Little, C (2007) *Hobbs' food poisoning and food hygiene*, 7th edn. Hodder Arnold, London.

Montville, TJ (2008) *Food microbiology*, 2nd edn. Wiley-Blackwell, Oxford.

Ray, B and Bhunia, A (2008) *Fundamental food microbiology*, 4th edn. CRC Press, Boca Raton, FL.

Weblinks

http://www. microbiologyonline. org. uk
This website is supported by the UK Society for General Microbiology and contains a wealth of information for students and teachers. There are images, videos, posters and podcasts, as well as suggestions for simple microbiology practicals suitable for both schoolchildren and university students.

The American Society of Microbiology supports two useful websites:
http://www. microbeworld. org/ for hundreds of images, videos, podcasts and news stories about microbiology for a general audience, and

http://www. microbelibrary. org/ for standard microbiology laboratory protocols including images, videos and animations intended for science educators.

http://www. cellsalive. com/howbig. htm
This popular commercial website includes an interactive video about cell sizes starting with a human hair and finishing with a virus.

Many university departments or individual academics produce inspirational websites about microbiology. These are useful but always check when the website was last updated. Academics move on to new jobs, retire or simply run out of steam or time to update their sites. Basic microbiological techniques like the Gram stain don't change but old news stories about outbreaks, scientific discoveries or legislation can be misleading unless placed correctly in their historical context.

http://www. shs. mmu. ac. uk/microbiology/
This website contains several useful videos of basic microbiological techniques, including Gram staining. The videos were produced by academics at a UK university and are intended for both students and teachers.

http://learn. genetics. utah. edu/content/begin/cells/scale/
This is an interactive exercise on cell sizes and scales supported by the University of Utah, USA. It starts with a coffee bean and works its way down in size through a grain of salt, a skin cell, baker's yeast, *E. coli*, various viruses, a water molecule and finally a carbon atom.

http://www. microbiologybytes. com
This website is managed by Dr Alan Cann, a virologist at the University of Leicester, UK. The site contains a wealth of images and podcasts about microbiology including videos of the Gram-staining technique.

3

Microbes are all around us

The limitations of microscopy

We can't see microorganisms but they are all around us, in air, water, soil, food, on dishcloths and chopping boards, as well as on human skin. In Chapter 2, we've seen how microscopes can be used to visualize these tiny creatures so that we can study their anatomy more closely. But microscopy is suitable only if large numbers of microbes are present and they are not hidden from view by bigger particles. Thus, inspecting samples of food or soil directly under the microscope is unlikely to reward us with clear images of all the microorganisms within them.

There are a number of other problems with microscopy as a tool for studying microorganisms. First, it cannot distinguish between live and dead microbes and tells us very little about their physiology and life cycle. An image of a microbe, like a picture of the human body, does not explain how the living organism works. Second, microscopy is relatively crude and cannot be used to identify microbes down to species level. Identifying the correct species in a food-poisoning investigation is as important as finding the real criminal in a human crime scene investigation.

In this chapter, we explore how the many bacteria, yeasts and moulds in the air, on surfaces and on our bodies can be studied using methods other than microscopy.

Microbes in the air

Figure 3.1 shows an example of the types of microbes that can be grown from the air using microbiological **growth media**. Microbes, like humans, need water and nutrients (food) to grow and multiply. General purpose growth media such as nutrient broth are made much like bouillon soup or stock, by boiling meat and bones to extract the proteins from them. Many microbes are happy to grow in their millions in these soups but some are fussy and require the addition of yeast extract, blood or milk to the basic broth to grow. Liquid media can be made into semi-solid gels by the addition of 1.5 per cent **agar**, a **carbohydrate** extracted from seaweed. All microbiological media are sterilized in autoclaves or pressure cookers to remove all possible contaminants prior to use.

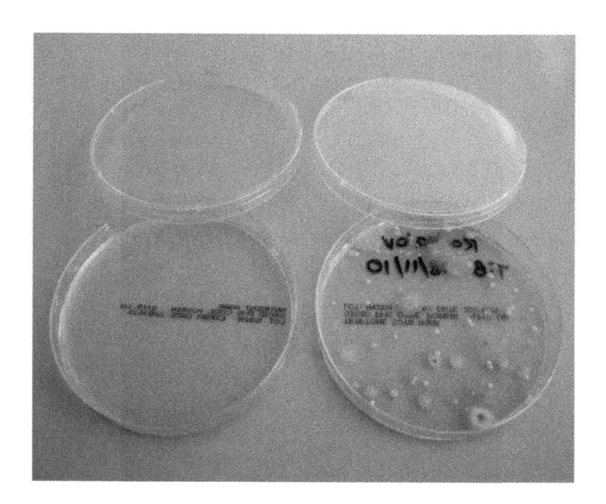

Figure 3.1 Air microbes growing on general purpose media. The Nutrient Agar plate on the right was left uncovered on a worktop in a busy kitchen for 2 hours to allow invisible bacteria and fungi in the air to settle on the surface of the agar. After incubation at 30°C overnight, the bacteria formed small cream and yellow colonies whilst moulds formed the large fluffy colonies. The sterile plate on the left remained covered throughout this period and is shown for comparison.

Sterile, agar-containing media are dispensed while hot and liquid in round, shallow dishes of 10 cm diameter. These are known as Petri dishes (Fig. 3.1), named after the scientist who developed them in Robert Koch's laboratory (see Box 3.1). Once cooled, the agar provides a large, flat surface area rich in nutrients for microbes to grow on. When spread on this surface and incubated for an appropriate

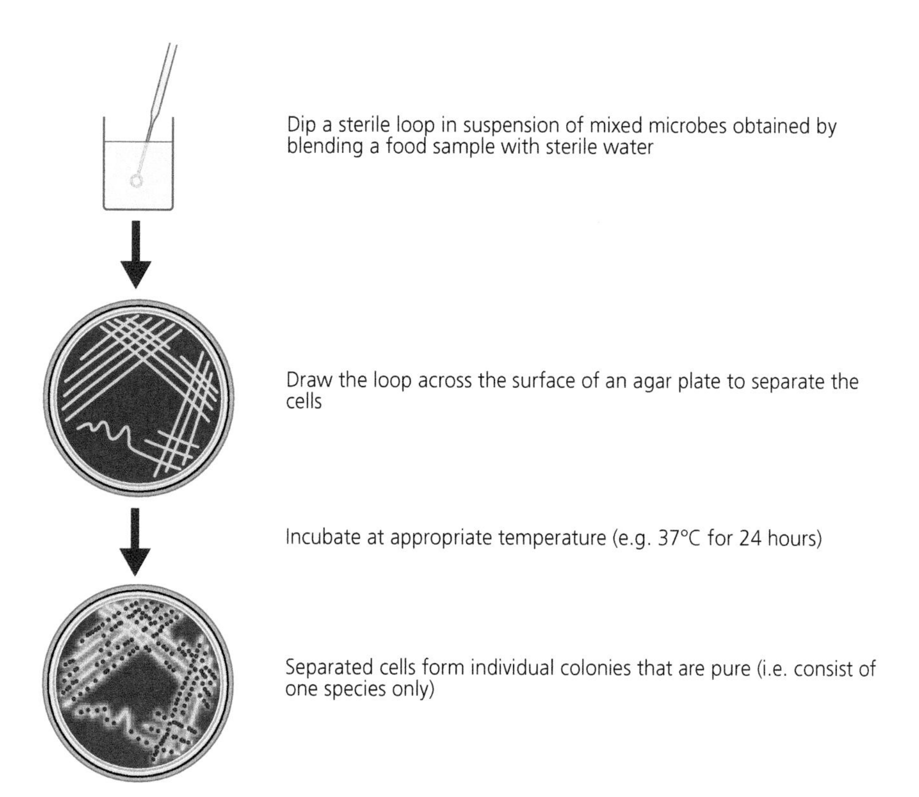

Figure 3.2 The 'streaking out' technique is used routinely to isolate individual microbial species from mixed populations.

Box 3.1 Microbiology Hall of Fame: Koch, the Hesses and Petri (late nineteenth century)

Many of the techniques used to this day for isolating and growing bacteria in culture were developed in Robert Koch's laboratory in the late nineteenth century. As a medical doctor, Koch was interested in infectious diseases and their causes. He suspected that specific bacteria might be responsible for causing diseases such as anthrax or tuberculosis but almost all specimens collected from sick patients or diseased animals were mixtures of microbes. It was impossible to tell which one had caused the illness.

Having noticed that a boiled potato left in the open air for a few days developed small dark spots, Koch decided to examine the spots under the microscope. He noticed that each spot had just one type of microbe in it and this gave him the idea that growing microbes on solid surfaces could be a useful way of isolating pure cultures. He went on to develop the technique of smearing sterile boiled slices of potato with specimens from diseased animals or patients and incubating them in a warm room until the appearance of pure colonies. By testing these pure cultures on animals, he was able to demonstrate that *Bacillus anthracis* is the cause of anthrax.

But the humble potato was not the ideal way of cultivating microbes, as some bacteria refused to grow on it altogether. Bacteria grew well on beef broth solidified with gelatin but its 'melt-in-the-mouth' properties so valued by chefs meant that the semi-solid media would liquefy on hot summer days and so ruin the experiment. Even on cooler days, some bacteria were able to digest gelatin, turning the semi-solid platforms into cloudy liquids overnight.

In 1880, Walther Hesse joined Koch's team. Walther's wife Angelina Fannie often assisted him in the laboratory and provided illustrations for his scientific papers. When Walther complained about his troubles with gelatin, Fannie suggested trying another gelling agent, agar-agar (now known simply as agar). She had learned about agar, an extract from red seaweed, from a neighbour who had lived for a while on the Indonesian island of Java. Like many modern-day chefs, Fannie used agar to make jellies and puddings that maintained their shape even on hot days. Walther added agar to beef broth and dispensed it in shallow dishes developed by another co-worker in Koch's lab, Julius Richard Petri. And so the agar plate, the workhorse of the microbiology laboratory to this day, was born.

Using all these techniques, Koch went on to isolate *Mycobacterium tuberculosis*, the causative agent of tuberculosis. There followed a golden age of classical microbiology, lasting about 40 years, when most of the major disease-causing bacteria were isolated.

time (often overnight) and at a suitable temperature (e.g. 37°C for many bacteria, 30°C for many fungi), microbes multiply to many millions of cells and form a colony that is visible to the naked eye.

Agar plates make it possible to separate mixed populations of microbes into their individual types by **streaking out**. This technique is shown in Fig. 3.2. The appearance of colonies, including their diameter (measured in millimetres), colour, form (smooth, rough or mucoid), opacity (transparent or opaque) and texture (dry or viscous) can be useful in identifying some microbes to species level.

Over the years, microbiologists have developed an arsenal of culture media to study microorganisms. **Selective media** contain ingredients that stop some species from growing but stimulate others to grow and multiply. For example, as shown in Fig. 3.3, malt extract agar is more acidic than nutrient agar and so encourages the more acid-tolerant yeasts and moulds to grow while bacteria, which are more sensitive to acids, are inhibited or grow more slowly. An even more selective agar is shown in Fig. 3.4. In this example, the chemical composition of the agar medium stimulates *Salmonella* to produce creamy-pink colonies with a black centre. All other bacteria deposited on this agar produce atypical, creamy colonies or do not grow at all.

Agar plates can also be used to work out the number of microbes present in a water or food sample. The number of colonies on a plate grown from a specified volume or weight of water/food can be used to calculate the number of **colony-forming units per millilitre (cfu/mL)** or **colony-forming units per gram (cfu/g)**. Microbial numbers in foods are discussed in more detail in Chapter 8.

The microbiological quality of air in a food preparation environment can be assessed by exposing agar plates to the atmosphere for a fixed period of time,

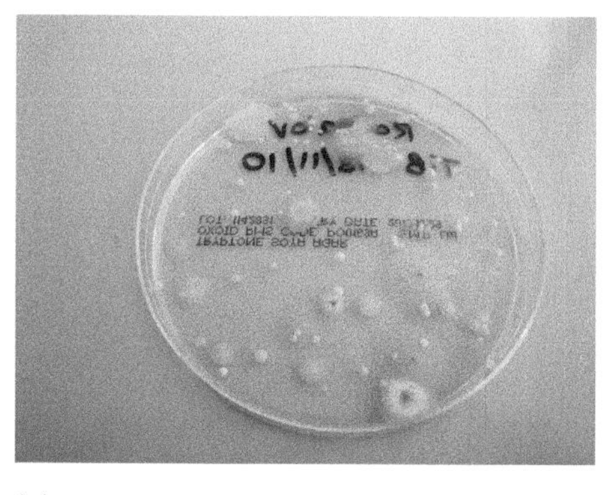

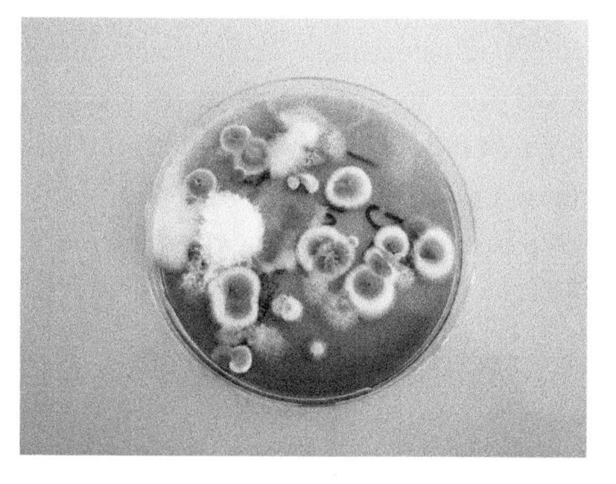

(a) **(b)**

Figure 3.3 Air microbes growing on general and selective media. The general-purpose tryptone soya agar (TSA) plate (a) and the selective malt extract agar (MEA) plate (b) were left uncovered, side-by-side, on a worktop for 2 hours. After incubation at 30°C overnight, more moulds grew on MEA, which is acidic, than on TSA, which is pH neutral.

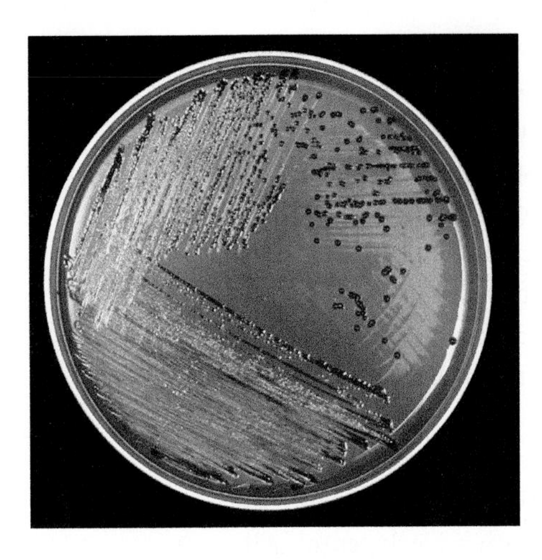

Figure 3.4 *Salmonella* spp. growing on a selective agar. The agar contains xylose lysine deoxycholate (XLD), which stimulate *Salmonella* to produce black colonies with a creamy-pink halo around them. Other bacteria do not grow on this agar or they produce colonies that lack the black centre. Figure courtesy of Centers for Disease Control and prevention (CDC).

incubating at an appropriate temperature and counting the number of colonies that have grown on the agar. This is a fairly simple technique but is biased towards heavier particles, for example yeasts and moulds tend to settle more quickly than bacteria. More accurate estimates of air quality can be made using mechanical air samplers that draw measured volumes of air through a slit and deposit the particles more evenly on the agar surface.

Microbes on inert surfaces

If microbes are in the air we breathe, it will come as no surprise that they can also be found on all surfaces around us.

Microbes in their millions have been isolated from toilet surfaces, drains and rubbish tips but it may not be so obvious that thousands of microbes can also be present on surfaces of seemingly clean, everyday objects. For example, the computer keyboard and electronic mouse are a magnet for microbes from dust particles and human hands. Eating your lunch while using your computer doesn't help either; at night, mice emerge from their hiding places to feast on the crumbs between the keys, leaving their droppings as a souvenir.

Microbes have been isolated from many other everyday objects, for example:

- grab rails on trains and buses;
- handbags and rucksacks;
- handles (on doors, cupboards, lockers, windows, shopping baskets);
- keypads and touchscreens for cash and ticket machines;
- electrical switches (for lights, fans, radiators);
- lift (elevator) buttons;

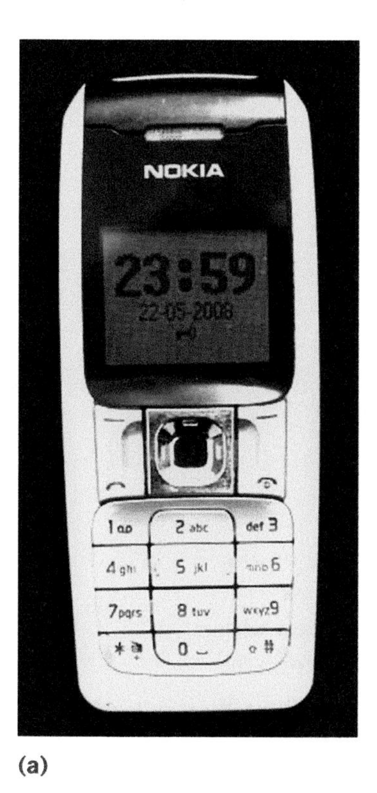

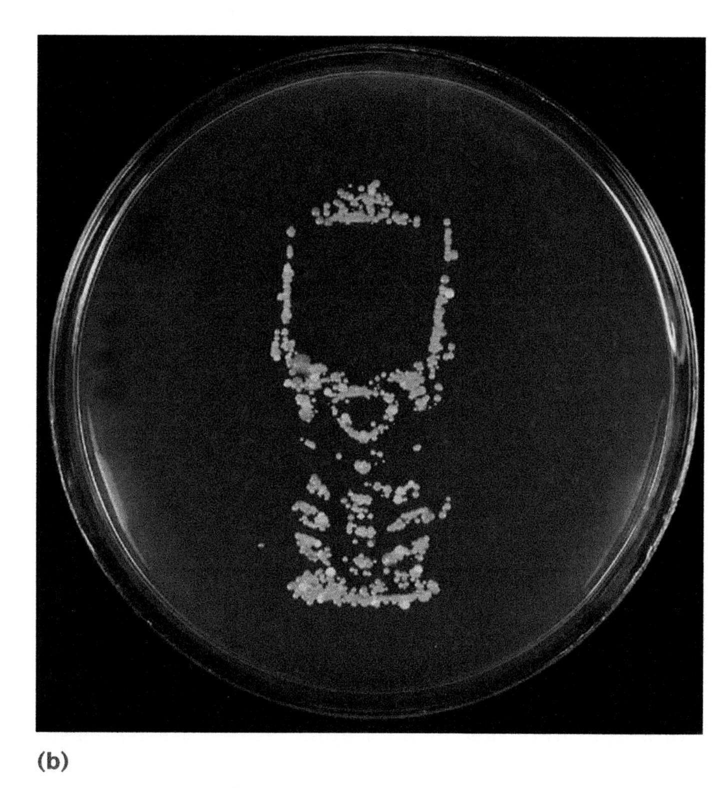

(a) (b)

Figure 3.5 Mobile phone and microbial colonies arising from its imprint on an agar plate. Figure courtesy of Professor Joanna Verran, Manchester Metropolitan University, Manchester, UK.

- remote controls (for TVs and other electrical equipment);
- pens;
- telephones (see mobile phone in Fig. 3.5);
- money (coins and notes);
- sink taps (kitchen and bathroom);
- sinks (kitchen and bathroom);
- soap dispensers.

In addition to the above, surfaces in kitchens often have microbes attached to them, for example:

- touchpads/controls for appliances (e.g. microwave and conventional ovens);
- all handles (e.g. fridges, cupboards, doors);
- cleaning sponges, cloths and brushes (especially when damp);

- dishcloths and towels (especially when damp);
- floor mops;
- staff clothing, uniforms, aprons;
- chopping boards made from all materials, including wood and plastics;
- mixing bowls (e.g. glass, ceramic, plastic);
- utensils, all tools with handles (e.g. knives);
- delicatessen slicers;
- work surfaces made of granite, marble and stainless steel;
- waste bins;
- papers and charts (e.g. recipes, cookbooks, food orders);
- any sites where dust is allowed to settle.

Swabbing, illustrated in Figs 3.6 and 3.7, is the basic technique used to assess the level of contamination or cleanliness of surfaces. The technique works best with flat, smooth surfaces. The method relies on effective removal of microbes from the surface and efficient transfer on to growth media. If done incorrectly or sloppily, it can lead to unreliable or misleading results. If used consistently, the results of swabbing can show trends and identify the need for improved cleaning and disinfection. This is discussed in more detail in Chapter 8.

Many surfaces lack food and moisture and so represent a relatively harsh environment for microbes to survive on. Nevertheless, bacteria such as *Staphylococcus aureus* and *Escherichia coli* can survive for several months on dry

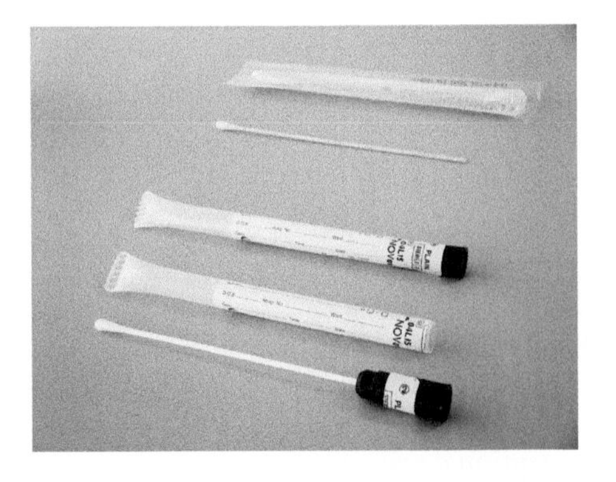

Figure 3.6 Examples of typical cotton wool swabs used to assess microbial contamination of all kinds of surfaces, including human skin.

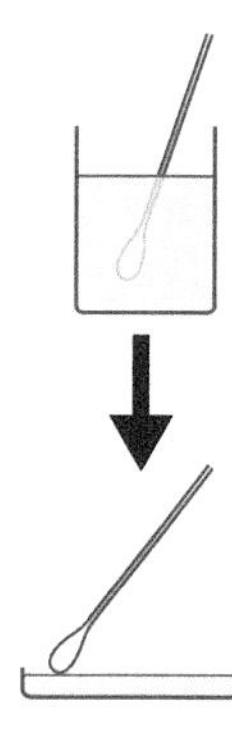

For dry surfaces, moisten sterile swab with sterile water. If surface is already moist, use dry swab

Swab a surface area of 10 by 10 cm twice at right angles to transfer microbes from the surface to the swab

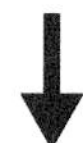

Streak out on appropriate agar plate and incubate at 30° or 37°C. Alternatively, break swab into sterile water, shake and use suspension to determine the number of organisms present

Figure 3.7 The swabbing technique is used to assess the level of microbial contamination on surfaces.

surfaces. Some *Salmonella* species have been recovered from surfaces more than 4 years after the initial contamination event.

Many microbes can survive stressful environmental conditions because of their ability to stick to surfaces and form **biofilms**. External structures, such as flagella and pili (see Chapter 2), help bacteria to make the initial contact with a surface. Once attached, microbes can multiply to form large communities of cells, stuck together and protected from the vagaries of the environment by a slimy coat of **polysaccharide**. These biofilms are sophisticated structures within which bacteria 'talk' to each other by secreting small signalling molecules. This form of communication between bacteria is known as **quorum sensing**.

Biofilms are important because they are more resistant to cleaning and disinfection than free-floating, individual microbial cells. Indeed, it has been shown that biofilms can survive treatment with disinfectants hundreds of times more concentrated than those needed to eliminate individual cells in suspensions. Control measures are discussed in more detail in Chapter 8.

Modern food-processing equipment is made of many different materials to which microbes can attach: stainless steel, glass, ceramic tiles, plastics, rubber, etc.

As a general rule, the rougher and more pitted a surface, the more likely it is that microbes can attach to it. However, the corollary does not apply. For example, *Salmonella* and *Listeria* attach readily to so-called 'non-stick' surfaces made of polytetrafluoroethylene (PTFE). It is difficult to predict the extent of microbial adhesion to any particular surface because the process depends not only on the nature of the surface but also on microbial species, temperature of the environment and the availability of water and nutrients (food).

It is normal practice in the food production and service industries to discard any food that has been dropped accidentally on the floor or other unsanitary surfaces. But how often are members of the public or untrained food handlers tempted to apply the 'five second rule' in the belief that if dropped food is picked up quickly enough, it is not too contaminated to consume? Research has shown that *Listeria monocytogenes* sticks to surfaces made of polypropylene (plastic), rubber, stainless steel and aluminium almost instantaneously. Similarly, *Salmonella* can be transferred from ceramic tiles, laminated wood and carpets to sliced bread and bologna sausage almost instantly. By the time you have bent down to pick up the dropped food, the damage has been done, so put the food in its rightful place: the waste bin!

Microbes on and in humans

It will be clear from the preceding sections that the human hand is a favourite mode of transportation for many microbes. So where do all these microbes originate?

The internal tissues and organs of a healthy person, such as the brain, blood and muscles, are normally free of microorganisms. However, the healthy human gut is teeming with microbes. The human digestive tract contains 10 times more bacteria than there are cells in the entire human body. Indeed, it could be argued that we are only part human because more than 90 per cent of the cells in our bodies are bacterial.

There are more than 800 different species of bacteria in the human **colon** (large intestine) and new ones are being discovered every year. Most of these microbes are not only harmless but are actually essential to our health and wellbeing. Without microbes in the gut, we could not digest our food properly. They help us to break down proteins and starches from our food, make vitamins such as B12 and K, regulate our immune system and prevent disease-causing bacteria from occupying the gut. Indeed, the gut is our most metabolically active organ but it could not function without the community of microbes within it.

The mix of microbes regularly found in a healthy gut is known as the normal **microflora**. When things go wrong with the balance of species in our gut, the whole body is affected. For example, a course of antibiotics can wipe out much of the normal intestinal flora, leading to diarrhoea. In such cases, many healthcare professionals now recommend a daily portion of a probiotic drink to replace the beneficial bacteria in the gut.

The market for **probiotics** has grown enormously since the 1990s. According to the World Health Organization (WHO), probiotics are defined as:

> 'live microorganisms which, when administered in adequate amounts, confer a health benefit on the host'.

The 'host' in this instance can be human or a farm animal. Probiotic drinks usually contain strains of *Lactobacillus* or *Bifidobacterium*.

Prebiotics are carbohydrate-based ingredients that stimulate the growth of beneficial strains already in the gut. Some food products can contain a combination of prebiotics and probiotics. These fermented milk drinks are intended to 'top up' the beneficial bacteria in the gut, particularly the lactobacilli and bifidobacteria.

The exact way in which probiotics influence health is not fully understood, partly due to our relatively scanty knowledge of the microbial ecosystem in our gut. However, this is likely to change in the next decade as the results of several large international research programmes become available. One example is the Human Microbiome Project, for which there is a weblink at the end of this chapter. These research projects will help us to unravel the microbial complexity in the gut and ultimately use the information to improve human health.

The faeces (solid wastes) of both humans and animals are a source of disease-causing microbes. The main way in which these microbes spread is known as the **faecal–oral route of transmission**, illustrated in Fig. 3.8. This mode of

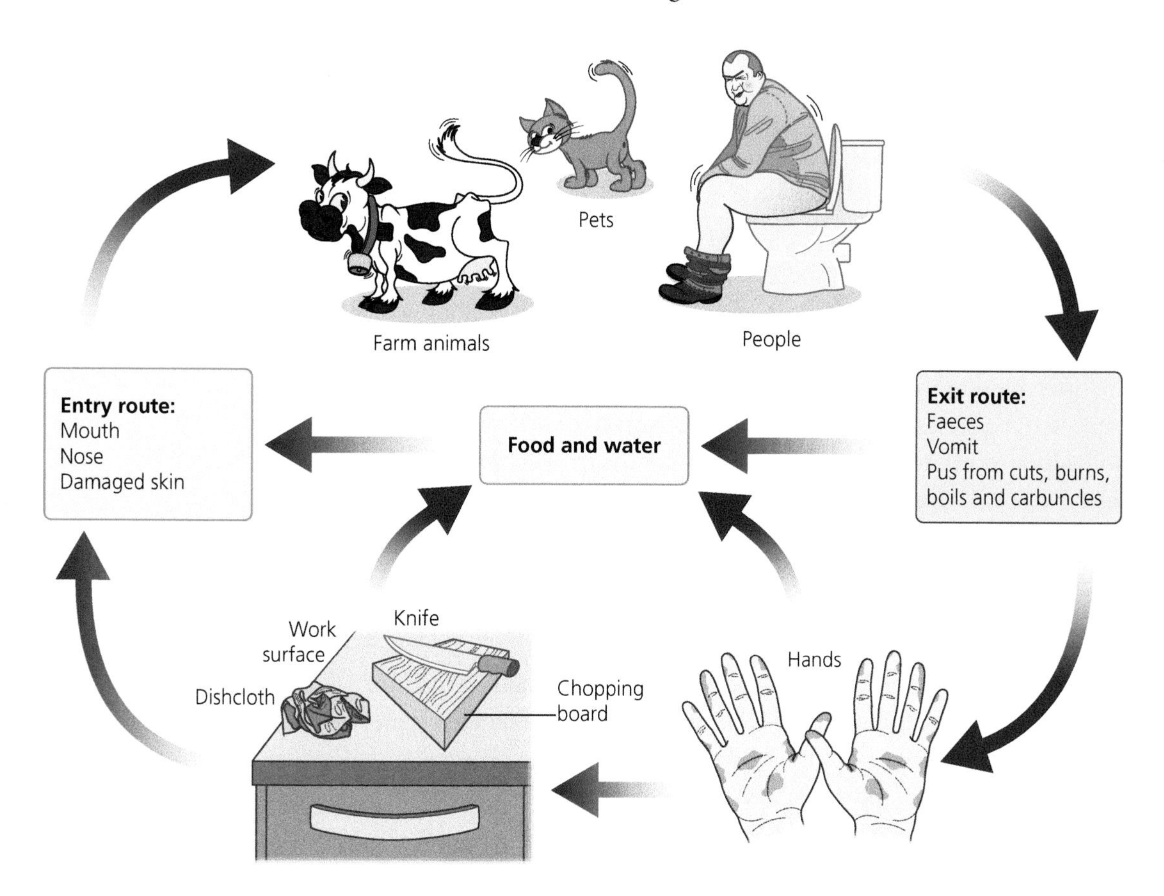

Figure 3.8 From turd to tongue. Many food-poisoning microbes are spread by the faecal–oral route.

transmission involves the ingestion of human or animal faeces through the mouth and is often mediated by human hands. Many food-poisoning microbes spread by the faecal–oral route.

By comparison with the gut, human skin is relatively sparsely populated with microbes. Conditions are drier and there are fewer nutrients for the microbes to grow on. Nevertheless, some of the more hardy bacteria such as *Staphylococcus*, *Propionibacterium* and *Corynebacterium* thrive on human skin. The propionibacteria are mainly responsible for the unsightly eruptions known as spots, zits, pimples and acne. *Staphylococcus epidermidis* is a common but harmless skin resident while its neighbour *Staphylococcus aureus* can cause food poisoning (more on this in Chapter 7).

Crime scene investigation: How are microbes identified?

The correct identification of microorganisms is crucial, not only for assessment of food hygiene and quality but also in investigations of food-poisoning incidents. The microbiologist is the equivalent of the forensic scientist in a crime scene investigation: both seek to identify the criminal, whether microbial or human. Unlike in TV dramas, however, it takes up to a week and often longer to correctly identify the perpetrator of the crime.

An example of a simplified scheme for identifying *Salmonella* in a food sample is shown in Table 3.1. Most foods contain a mixture of many different microbes and the first step in the identification of a suspected food-poisoning organism is to separate it from all the other microbes present. As *Salmonella* and other poisoners are often present in much lower numbers than other bacteria, the food sample is subjected to a series of enrichment steps designed to shift the growth of the mixed population towards a particular group of organisms. This is followed by plating on selective media (see Fig. 3.4) and biochemical testing of the typical colonies isolated. Since food-poisoning bacteria occur in many foods and the environment, identification to species level is often not enough and further confirmation of type or strain is also necessary. As shown in Table 3.1, it can take 4–9 days to confirm the presence of *Salmonella* in a food.

Like microscopy, culture-dependent methods have their limitations as tools for studying and identifying microbes. Growing microbes on agar plates is lengthy, laborious and expensive. Their cultivation requires specialist laboratories, complex equipment and teams of highly trained staff. By their very nature, culture-dependent methods are retrospective. By the time the presence of a food-poisoning microbe is confirmed, the organism in question may have wreaked havoc in a population and caused many cases of foodborne illness.

Table 3.1 Detecting and confirming the presence of *Salmonella* in food: a simplified example

Procedure	Time taken
Weigh 25 g of food; add to 225 ml of pre-enrichment medium (buffered peptone water); homogenize and incubate at 37°C for 16–20 hours	1 day
⬇ Take a sample of the above (e.g. 10 ml) and add to an enrichment medium (Rappaport–Vassiliadis broth or selenite–cystine broth); incubate at 37°C for 48 hours	1–2 days
⬇ At 24 hours and 48 hours, plate out the above on selective agar, e.g. xylose lysine deoxycholate (XLD) (see Fig. 3.4); incubate at 37°C for 24 hours (48 hours if necessary to obtain typical colonies)	1–2 days
⬇ Preliminary identification possible at this stage but must be confirmed by picking five characteristic colonies from each selective agar, transferring to nutrient agar and incubating at 37°C for 24 hours	1–4 days
⬇ Confirmation using biochemical, immunological and molecular techniques; interpretation of results	
Total time	4–9 days

Many scientists are working on developing more rapid methods to shorten the time required to correctly identify a microbe. Some of these techniques, known as **immunoassays**, involve the detection of specific microbial products such as proteins using antibodies. Others involve the analysis of the microbial DNA. Just like DNA fingerprinting of suspects in murder cases or paternity disputes, microbial DNA can be fingerprinted. The widespread adoption of molecular techniques and their ability to discriminate between strains within a species have made it possible to investigate large international outbreaks of food poisoning more rapidly and reliably. In the next chapter, we will look more closely at the extent of the food-poisoning problem from a global perspective.

Chapter 3 Quiz

1 Where can we find microbes?
2 What conditions do you think would encourage the growth of microbes?
3 If you exposed nutrient agar plates and malt extract agar plates to air, would you expect to see differences between them after incubation? If so, why?
4 Name five examples of inert surfaces on everyday objects that may have microbes on them.
5 Name a disease-causing microbe that can live on human skin and cause food poisoning.

Further reading

Willey, J, Woolverton, C and Sherwood, L (2008). *Prescott's Principles of Microbiology*, 8th edn. McGraw Hill. http://www.mcgraw-hill.co.uk/html/0071313672.html

The above textbook is intended for science students, so may be best attempted after you have finished reading this book. The accompanying laboratory manual *Laboratory Exercises in Microbiology* provides 65 laboratory practicals, some of which can be adapted for students interested in food.

Weblinks

The Wellcome Trust produces a wealth of reliable information on human health, food, nutrition and microbial diseases of all kinds. The information is intended for the general public and is always presented in an accessible format accompanied by beautiful illustrations, videos and podcasts. Many of the resources are available to download for free. A site well worth visiting is:
http://www. wellcome. ac. uk/Education-resources/index. htm

For images of microorganisms growing on agar plates or up close and personal (on the human body), visit the Public Health Image Library at the United States Centers for Disease Control and Prevention at:
http://phil. cdc. gov/phil/home. asp

For more images and multimedia files, visit this site, supported by the American Society of Microbiology:
http://www. microbelibrary. org/

For information about the UK Gut Week that takes place every August, visit:
http://www. loveyourgut. com/gut-week/

A regular news bulletin about probiotic research can be obtained from the *Science for Health* website intended for health professionals and sponsored by Yakult:
http://hcp. yakult. co. uk/

For more information on the Human Microbiome Project, visit:
https://commonfund. nih. gov/hmp/

Section II: Main Course

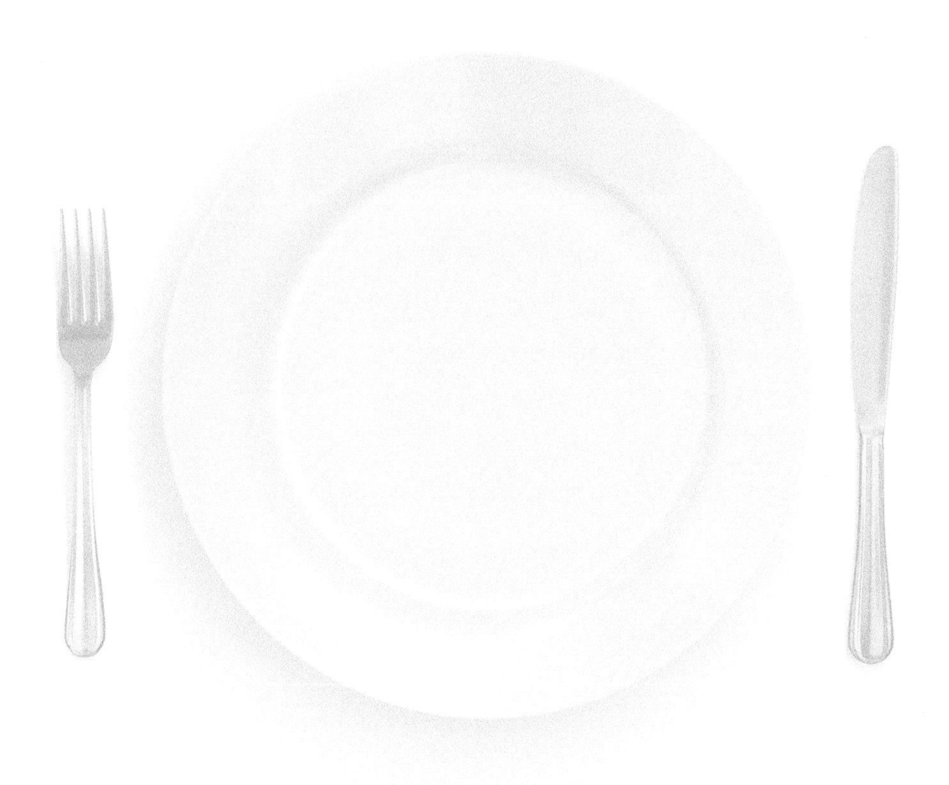

'Dans les champs de l'observation,
le hasard ne favorise que les esprits préparés. '
('In the field of observation,
chance favours only prepared minds')

Louis Pasteur,
developer of early forms of pasteurization, 1854

4

The global food-poisoning problem

There are many possible **hazards** (dangers) associated with food and drink and not all of them are of microbial origin. For example, there are *physical hazards* such as pieces of glass, metal or plastic that may be introduced accidentally during harvest and processing of foods. Bone fragments, fruit pips, wings of insects and even whole rats have been known to find their way into food. *Chemical hazards* can be present naturally, such as in poisonous mushrooms, or accidentally as in the migration of plasticizers from packaging into food. Chemical contamination of food can occur via seepage of agricultural chemicals (e.g. insecticides, herbicides, fungicides) through soil or from industrial effluents that may be high in lead, mercury or cadmium.

Although less common than in previous centuries, deliberate chemical adulteration of food still occurs occasionally. In 2008, a cattle farmer in eastern China sold a powder laced with melamine to a dairy producer who used it illegally to raise the protein content of watered-down milk. Melamine is a chemical normally used in the manufacture of plastics. The chemical causes liver damage, particularly in young children. By 2009, six infants were dead and another 300 000 people needed hospital treatment after consuming milk-based products laced with melamine. The company that supplied the contaminated baby formula was fined 50 million yuan (US$7.3 million or nearly £5 million), 60 people were arrested and more than 20 jailed, two for life. The farmer and original milk producer were both sentenced to death although their sentences were eventually changed to life imprisonment.

Physical and chemical contamination of foods, whether deliberate or accidental, is important but in terms of numbers of people affected, *biological hazards* are much more common. Biological hazards are organisms or by-products of organisms that can harm human health by causing infections, poisoning or allergies. In this book we are focusing on microbes as biological hazards and main agents of foodborne disease.

What is foodborne disease?

The World Health Organization (WHO) defines *foodborne disease* (or *foodborne illness*) as:

'any disease of an infectious or toxic nature caused by or thought to be caused by the consumption of food or water'.

The term *foodborne disease* is broad and includes a wide variety of symptoms throughout the human body. A related term, *food poisoning*, is narrower and is associated with illnesses causing gut symptoms, such as diarrhoea. However, in practice, the two terms are often used interchangeably. In common with other textbooks, the term food poisoning is used in this book in its broadest sense and includes all foodborne diseases, irrespective of symptoms.

Those microbes that cause illness in humans, animals or plants are known as **pathogens**. The foodborne illnesses caused by these microbial agents can be divided into two types:

- **Infections**: the microbes multiply in the human body, usually in the intestinal tract (gut), to cause illness.
- Intoxications: the microbes produce toxins (poisons) in food or during passage through the human intestinal tract. It is the toxins rather than the microbes themselves that cause the illness. Toxins that affect the gut are known as **enterotoxins** while those that affect the nervous system are known as **neurotoxins**.

Some examples of microbial infections and intoxications are shown in Box 4.1.

Box 4.1 Microbial causes of foodborne disease

Bacteria that cause infections
e.g. *Campylobacter jejuni*, *Listeria monocytogenes*, *Salmonella* spp.

Bacteria that produce toxins (poisons)
e.g. *Staphylococcus aureus* produces an enterotoxin; *Clostridium botulinum* produces a neurotoxin

Algae
e.g. paralytic poisoning from shellfish that accumulate toxins from algae

Fungi (moulds)
e.g. mycotoxins (fungal poisons) produced by *Aspergillus* and *Penicillium* spp.

Viruses
e.g. norovirus, hepatitis A

Protozoa
e.g. *Entamoeba histolytica*, *Giardia lamblia*, *Cryptosporidium parvum*

The minimum number of microbes needed to cause disease is known as the **infective dose**. The infective dose for any specific organism is difficult to measure. Published figures are often rough estimates based on retrospective analysis of foods that are known to have caused illness and experiments with healthy volunteers. An individual's susceptibility to any given infective dose depends on age and state of health. The infective dose can also depend on the food in which the microbes are eaten. For example, fatty foods can protect microbes from the damaging effects of stomach acids, increasing the likelihood of infection.

The most common symptoms of food poisoning are diarrhoea and abdominal pain (cramps). These are sometimes accompanied by fever and/or vomiting. These symptoms are commonly referred to as **gastroenteritis**. This term is somewhat misleading, as foodborne illness rarely involves the stomach (*gastro-*) but is more usually associated with the small and large intestine (*-enteritis*). Many foodborne pathogens can produce symptoms that are much more severe than gastroenteritis. Further details about these are given in Chapters 5–7.

When discussing food-poisoning statistics, the terms **case**, **outbreak** and **sporadic case** are often used. These are defined below:

- A **case**: a microorganism is isolated from a person with symptoms of a specific illness.
- An **outbreak**: there are two or more related cases.
- A **sporadic case**: the sick person has no known connection with another person infected with the same organism.

The size of the food-poisoning problem

The levels of foodborne disease are unacceptably high. There are millions of cases of foodborne illness reported every year in the developed world, leading to tens of thousands of hospitalizations and several thousand deaths. Some examples of food-poisoning statistics for three countries are shown in Table 4.1. In addition, the costs to society in terms of medical services and lost productivity at work are measured in billions of pounds, dollars or euros. In the developing world, the numbers are even higher.

Although numbers vary from country to country and from region to region, the World Health Organization (WHO) estimates that unsafe food sickens one in three people every year.

Not only is the burden of disease large across the world, but the numbers of some foodborne diseases appear to be increasing. For example, campylobacteriosis (caused by *Campylobacter* spp.) and yersiniosis (caused by *Yersinia* spp.) are showing upward trends in Europe (Table 4.2). The overall incidence of many common foodborne illnesses in the USA has changed very little in the period between 2005 and 2010. In the UK, a substantial downward trend in foodborne illness recorded between 2000 and 2004 has since been reversed and the numbers of cases in 2009 were nearly as high as those reported a decade earlier.

To place some of these figures in context, the number of cases of foodborne illness reported in the UK is about four times higher than that of non-fatal road traffic injuries. In order to operate a car or other motorized vehicle legally, most countries require drivers to pass a stringent test and acquire a licence permitting them to drive. Driving without a licence is illegal. There is no equivalent requirement for food handlers. Although food premises in many countries need to be registered, there is no licensing based on competence in preparing food safely.

Table 4.1 Foodborne illness in three countries of the developed world (data from US Centers for Disease Control and Prevention (CDC); UK and Australian Food Standards Agencies, 2010)

Country	Number per year			Estimated cost (health care, lost work and disability)
	Cases of illness	People hospitalized	Deaths	
Australia	5.4 million	18 000	120	A$1.3 billion
UK	1 million	20 000	500	£1.5 billion
USA	48 million	128 000	3 000	US$152 billion

Table 4.2 General trends and number of cases reported for main food- and waterborne diseases in 31 European countries (population 501 million) (data from European Centre for Disease Prevention and Control, 2010)

Disease (causative agent)	General trend	Number of cases notified per 100 000 population
Mainly foodborne		
Campylobacteriosis (*Campylobacter* spp.)	⇧	44.1
Vero/Shiga toxin-producing *Escherichia coli* (VTEC/STEC)	⇔	0.7
Hepatitis A	⇩	3.3
Listeriosis (*Listeria monocytogenes*)	⇔	0.3
Salmonellosis (*Salmonella* spp.)	⇩	29.8
Yersiniosis (*Yersinia enterocolitica*)	⇧	2.7
Mainly waterborne		
Cryptosporidiosis (*Cryptosporidium* spp.)	⇔	2.4
Giardiasis (*Giardia lamblia*)	⇩	59.6
Shigellosis (*Shigella* spp.)	⇔	1.8

Foodborne poisoning: the tip of the iceberg

Many foodborne illnesses are not reported to public health authorities and so are not counted in official statistics. A person suffering from foodborne illness may experience relatively mild symptoms and so not visit a doctor. Even if the sick person seeks medical care, the doctor may make a tentative diagnosis on the basis of symptoms and not report the illness to the public health authorities. As shown in Table 4.3, the symptoms of many foodborne illnesses are so similar that they cannot be used to make a definitive diagnosis. Unless the doctor takes a faeces (stool) sample from the patient and sends it to a laboratory for analysis, the pathogen causing the illness will never be confirmed.

Some examples of large outbreaks are shown in Table 4.4. But for every large outbreak, there are likely to be many times the number of sporadic cases that have not been reported and so are undetected.

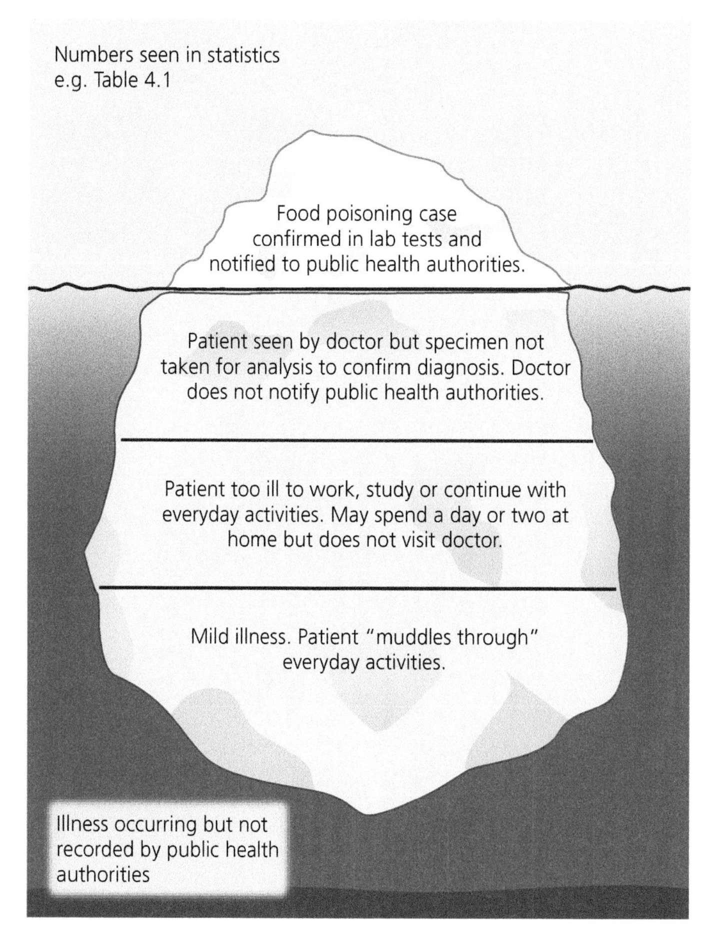

Figure 4.1 Food-poisoning statistics are just the tip of the iceberg. The ratio of notified cases to those experiencing mild symptoms is estimated to be anywhere between 1:135 and 1:1500.

Table 4.3 Time of onset, symptoms, cause and duration of foodborne illness

Time from eating food to onset of symptoms	Typical symptoms	Cause of illness		Usual duration of illness
		Microbe/toxin	Main foods affected	
1 hour or less	Facial swelling and flushing, skin rashes, itching, nausea, vomiting, headache, dizziness, anaphylactic shock	Allergic reactions	Nuts, eggs, milk, wheat, monosodium glutamate, histamine in tuna fish	Less than 1 day to several days
as above	Nausea, vomiting, abdominal pain and neurologic symptoms such as blurred vision, dizziness, paralysis	Fish and shellfish toxins	Fish and shellfish	Several days
as above	Nausea, vomiting and abdominal pain	*Bacillus cereus* (vomiting type) toxin	Boiled and fried rice	1 day
2–6 hours	Nausea, vomiting, abdominal pain and diarrhoea but no fever	*Staphylococcus aureus* toxin	Meat and poultry, dairy products, cream cakes, cooked fish and seafoods	1 day
8–20 hours	Abdominal pain, diarrhoea, sometimes nausea	*Bacillus cereus* (diarrhoeal type)	Meat products, soups, sauces	1 day
as above	Diarrhoea, abdominal pain, nausea but rarely vomiting	*Clostridium perfringens*	Cooked meat and poultry	1 day
12–36 hours	Disturbed vision, difficulty in speaking and swallowing. Progressive weakness and respiratory failure	*Clostridium botulinum*	Home-canned foods. Vacuum-packed fish and other seafoods	Slow recovery over 6–8 months
12–72 hours	Watery diarrhoea and pain or prolonged diarrhoea with blood in stool	Verotoxigenic *Escherichia coli*	Raw beef and other red meat, cooked meats, fresh produce	1–7days

as above	Vomiting, diarrhoea, abdominal pain and fever	*Salmonella* spp.	Poultry (chicken, turkey, duck), meat, raw milk, fresh produce	2–7 days
as above	as above	*Shigella*	Water or fresh produce irrigated with contaminated water	2–7 days
as above	as above	*Vibrio parahaemolyticus*	Raw and cooked fish and seafoods (prawns, crabs)	2–5 days
as above	as above	*Yersinia enterocolitica*	Milk and dairy products, raw pork	1–2 weeks
1–2 days	Vomiting, diarrhoea, abdominal pain and fever	Norovirus	Oysters and other shellfish	1–2 days
2–11 days	Flu-like symptoms, abdominal pain, severe diarrhoea, cramps and nausea, fever	*Campylobacter jejuni*	Poultry, raw milk and untreated water	Up to 3 weeks
1–70 days (usually 1–8 days)	Flu-like symptoms, meningitis, encephalitis (brain fever), septicaemia (blood poisoning), miscarriage, stillbirth	*Listeria monocytogenes*	Soft cheeses, pâté, deli meats	Weeks/ months
1–6 weeks	Abdominal pain, diarrhoea, headache, drowsiness, ulcers	*Entamoeba histolytica*	Water or fresh produce irrigated with contaminated water	Few days to a month
as above	Abdominal pain, mucoid diarrhoea, weight loss	*Giardia lamblia*	as above	
1 week	Watery diarrhoea	*Cyclospora cayetanensis*	as above	
15–50 days	Nausea, abdominal pain, tiredness, jaundice	Hepatitis	Water or fresh produce irrigated with contaminated water	Weeks to months

Table 4.4 Examples of large food-poisoning outbreaks

Year	Country	Number of cases	Food	Cause
1994	USA	224 000	Ice cream	*Salmonella* Enteritidis
1996	Japan	7000	Bean sprouts served to school children	Verotoxin-producing *Escherichia coli* O157:H7
2000	Canada	2300	Drinking water	Verotoxin-producing *Escherichia coli* O157 and *Campylobacter*
2005	Spain	2138	Precooked vacuum-packed roast chicken	*Salmonella* Hador
2008	USA	1400	Jalapeno peppers imported from Mexico	*Salmonella* St Paul
2011	Germany and France	4178	Sprouted fenugreek seeds imported from Egypt	Verotoxin-producing *Escherichia coli* O104:H4

It would be impossible to calculate the exact ratio of foodborne illness in the community for every laboratory-confirmed case reported to public health authorities. However, as shown in Fig. 4.1, the number of cases in the community is likely to be several hundred times the number of those reported. Estimates of the ratio of reported to mild illness vary from 1:135 to 1:1500.

Why is food poisoning such a big problem?

Modern food production is hugely complex and safety problems can arise at any stage of the chain: on the farm, during transportation and distribution, at the food processing factory or the retailer, during foodservice or in the consumer's home. A food product purchased from the supermarket or a dish ordered in a restaurant may contain ingredients from all over the world.

In the following paragraphs, we examine the reasons why foodborne disease is so common and why some pathogens seem to be a growing problem.

Improved surveillance

> 'Good surveillance does not necessarily ensure the making of the right decisions but it reduces the chances of wrong ones.'
>
> *Alexander Langmuir 1963*

Surveillance is the systematic collection of data, analysis and tracking of the main infectious diseases, including foodborne illness. A reliable surveillance programme is not just an academic exercise. Good surveillance underpins public health policy and is essential for developing evidence-based control measures.

Some of the recent increases in foodborne illness could probably be attributed to our improved ability to detect and track infectious diseases across the globe. We are getting better at measuring the burden of foodborne disease. However, the data are patchy and many countries of the world lack good surveillance programmes. Even the best national surveillance systems miss the majority of cases of foodborne disease as seen in Fig. 4.1.

Good global surveillance is crucial, not only to detect foodborne illness but also to provide early warning and hopefully stop emerging outbreaks before they grow too big. Figure 4.2 shows how an early reporting and rapid response system can reduce the numbers of cases of foodborne disease in an outbreak.

Some of the authorities involved in surveillance and rapid alerting are shown in Box 4.2.

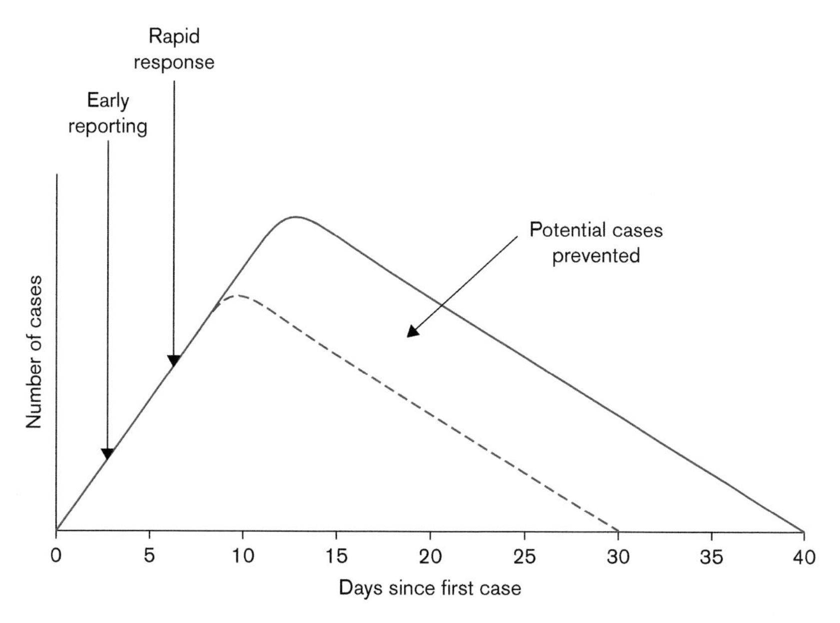

Figure 4.2 A typical outbreak curve showing the number of cases with (----) and without (——) early reporting and rapid response systems in place. In an outbreak caused by a common source such as food or water, there is a rapid increase up to a peak and then a more gradual decline in cases of illness. If the illness can also spread from person to person, the tail of the curve can be longer.

Population growth and intensive farming

The world's human population is growing relentlessly. In the past 40 years of the twentieth century, the numbers of people on Earth doubled from 3 to 6 billion.

Box 4.2 Examples of surveillance programmes and networks

Global

- The *International Food Safety Authorities Network (INFOSAN)* is a joint initiative between the World Health Organization (WHO) and the Food and Agriculture Organization of the United Nations (FAO). This global network includes 177 member states. Information on food safety is shared and collaboration between countries is promoted. For more information, visit: http://www.who.int/foodsafety/fs_management/infosan/en/index.html
- Every country member of INFOSAN appoints a designated emergency contact point for communications during urgent events. These contact points form the *Global Outbreak Alert and Response Network (GOARN)*. For more information, visit: http://www.who.int/csr/outbreaknetwork/en/
- Help is available for countries that need to strengthen their capacity to detect, control and prevent foodborne infections through the *Global Foodborne Infections Network (GFN)*. This was formerly known as the Global Salm-Surv (GSS) and was initially set up to focus on *Salmonella* surveillance. The network now has a wider scope and includes *Escherichia coli* and *Campylobacter* spp. The network has over 1000 laboratory members. For more information, visit: http://www.who.int/gfn/en/index.html
- The *WHO Foodborne Epidemiology Reference Group (FERG)* was established in 2007 to estimate the global burden of foodborne disease. FERG is a group of internationally renowned experts in a range of subjects relevant to foodborne disease epidemiology. For more information, visit: http://www.who.int/foodsafety/foodborne_disease/ferg/en/index3.html

European

- The *European Centre for Disease Prevention and Control (ECDC)* manages the surveillance network for human gastrointestinal infections in 31 European countries. Previously known as EnterNet, the focus of surveillance is now on *Salmonella* spp., Shiga-toxin producing *E. coli* (STEC), *Campylobacter* spp. and antibiotic resistance patterns across Europe. For more information, visit: http://ecdc.europa.eu
- The European Union (EU) *Rapid Alert System for Food and Feed (RASFF)* provides weekly news of border alerts and food recalls for products imported into the EU and distributed within the EU. The system covers both microbial and chemical contamination. For more information, visit: http://ec.europa.eu/food/food/rapidalert/index_en.htm

USA

- The extensive *FoodNet* programme managed by the US *Centers for Disease Control and Prevention (CDC)* collects data on the incidence of *Campylobacter, Salmonella*, verotoxin-producing *E coli, Shigella, Listeria monocytogenes, Vibrio, Yersinia, Cryptosporidium* and *Cyclospora*. For more information, visit: http:www.cdc.gov/foodborneburden and http://www.cdc.gov/FoodNet

Currently at 7 billion, the world population is predicted to reach 9 billion by 2044 and 10 billion by the end of this century (United Nations and US Census Bureau data).

Farm animal populations have followed similar trends to those of humans. The numbers of cattle, pigs, chickens, ducks and farmed fish have increased proportionally to human numbers, with poultry and pigs predominating. Intensification of food production increases the risks of pathogen spread and persistence. Factors such as the improper use of manure, agricultural chemicals and contaminated water, confined animal housing and feeding, lack of appropriate storage and post-harvest handling, and a poorly trained and paid migrant work force, all contribute to food safety challenges.

Urbanization

The rate of migration from rural areas to cities accelerated in the late twentieth century. By 2010, more than half of the global population lived in cities. According to the United Nations, this trend is continuing and by 2030, 60 per cent of the world's population will live in cities or urban regions. City-bound migrants are also contributing to the growth in the number of megacities in which populations exceed 10 million. Of the 22 megacities currently in existence worldwide, 17 are in developing countries.

Continuing urbanization will have a serious environmental and public health impact, with pressures increasing on water supplies as well as on sanitation and waste disposal services. Industrialization and mass production of food can also lead to habitat encroachment. For example, more than half of the deforestation in the Amazon basin is for cattle ranching and growing animal feed crops.

Vulnerable populations

People respond differently to foodborne pathogens. Some may be infected without any outward signs of illness whereas others experience a range of symptoms from the very mild to the very severe or even death. It has been estimated that about one person in six belongs to a more vulnerable or 'at-risk' group in terms of susceptibility to infection from foodborne pathogens.

One of the most important factors influencing a person's vulnerability to foodborne disease is age (Fig. 4.3). Infants, young children and the elderly are more vulnerable to infection and once infected, suffer more serious symptoms of disease. This is a growing problem because the world has an ageing population. In the 25-year period before 2010, life expectancy in developed countries increased steadily so that people over 65 years old now represent nearly one fifth of the population in countries such as the UK, USA and Japan. By 2035, one third of the populations of Germany, Italy and Japan will be aged 65 years or over. The number

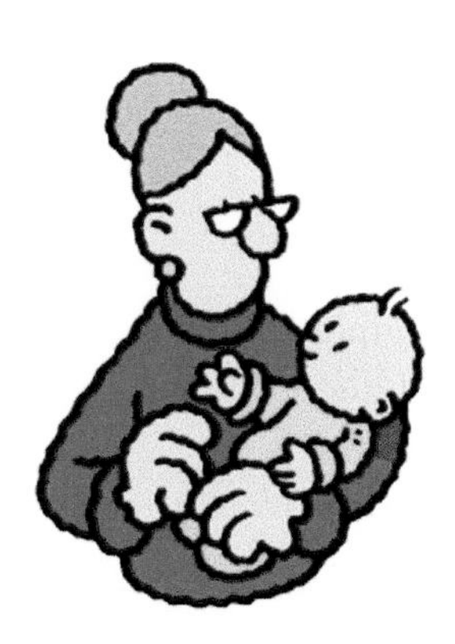

Figure 4.3 The elderly and young children are more vulnerable to infection, including food poisoning.

of centenarians is also growing. For example, the number of people aged over 100 years is expected to increase to around 420 000 in Japan and over half a million in Europe in the next two decades.

In addition to the elderly and the very young, there are other groups of people who are more vulnerable to foodborne disease:

- pregnant women and their unborn children;
- people with immune systems suppressed by medication or illness (e.g. cancer patients, HIV-positive individuals, diabetics, transplant patients);
- people on antacid medication;
- alcoholics and drug abusers;
- the malnourished (the sick, the homeless, people in long-term residential care)
- the undernourished (mainly in developing countries).

Increased mobility (of people and food)

As recently as the middle of the twentieth century, most consumers in the developed world either grew their own food in their garden or farm, or purchased it from small local producers. Fresh fruit and vegetables were available only when in season. Long-distance shipping and widespread international trade now make it possible to eat green beans from Kenya or mangoes from Mexico in the depths of the Northern winter. International trading in foods has transformed food-safety management from a local issue to a global public health problem.

People have also become more mobile. About 1 million people cross an international border every day. But diseases do not respect borders. By the time an infectious disease is detected, it is too late to close the borders. The extent to which humans and foods traverse the globe in a 24-hour period is vividly illustrated in a 2-minute video clip on YouTube showing air traffic across a world map (go to http://www. youtube. com and type in 'World air traffic in 24 hours').

Emerging pathogens and hazards

In the late 1970s, the successful implementation of mass vaccination programmes and widespread availability of effective antibiotics led some scientists to predict an imminent human victory over infectious diseases. In those days of heady optimism, I was advised by an eminent professor to abandon the microbiological theme of my Master's dissertation in public health. He commented scornfully that it would be all too easy to develop new control measures for bacterial contamination of drinking water and suggested that I should focus on something more challenging, such as cancer or heart disease. We know now that microbial control is far from easy and that infectious diseases are still very much with us. We may have won a few battles but the war rages on.

The speed with which microbes adapt and evolve ensures that as soon as one pathogen is under control, another one is likely to emerge. For example, the number of reported foodborne illnesses attributed to *Salmonella* spp. has decreased since its peak in the 1990s but the numbers of cases due to *Campylobacter jejuni* have increased. Old favourites have come back to haunt us but this time in their antibiotic-resistant form. For example, methicillin-resistant *Staphylococcus aureus* (MRSA) and *Clostridium difficile* are creating havoc in our hospitals. Bacteria such as *Legionella* and viruses such as HIV or severe acute respiratory virus (SARV) were largely unheard of before the 1980s but are now responsible for millions of cases of illness.

Advances in our understanding of well-known foodborne pathogens have also led to the recognition of new, emerging hazards. For example, recent outbreaks of salmonellosis associated with chocolate and peanut butter came as a surprise, as *Salmonella* cannot grow in low-moisture foods (further details in Chapter 5).

Changing lifestyles and consumer demands

Since the 1980s, consumers in the developed world have become more affluent, with increasing proportions of the household budget spent on catered meals and eating out. For example, the food service industry in the USA served 130 million meals per day in 2010, representing nearly half of the US food dollar expenditure. Ready-prepared meals that require brief reheating in a microwave oven were virtually unknown three decades ago, but the chillers used to display them now occupy increasing amounts of floor space in supermarkets. Catered meals require extensive handling and so the potential for the spread of disease increases. Furthermore, as less food is prepared and eaten in the home, so the skills of cooking and preparing foods safely by the individual are lost.

Consumer opposition to many food additives and demand for less heavily processed foods has meant that food manufacturers have fewer options for preserving foods. At the same time, trips to the supermarket to purchase food have become less frequent, creating an even greater challenge for food scientists to solve.

Nutritional recommendations to reduce intakes of saturated fats, refined carbohydrates and salt have also had an impact. For example, reduced levels of salt in 'sweetcure' bacon and sugar in jam mean that these products now require refrigeration whereas in the past they were stable at room temperature.

An explosion of new product development has contributed to the increased complexity of the food chain. There are now more potential vehicles for foodborne pathogens than ever before. For example, the fruit juice that was usually consumed in the morning and came from frozen concentrate is now consumed throughout the day in many forms. From smoothies to flavoured waters, these beverages can be made from exotic fruits such as pomegranate, mango or passion fruit, and are often enriched with vitamins, minerals and other ingredients claiming health benefits. Even water is no longer just tap water: it's bottled water sourced from 'natural' springs or mountains, carbonated or still, enriched with minerals or purified.

Other lifestyle factors may also contribute to the changing landscape of foodborne illness. These include increased exposure to ethnic foods through migration and holiday travel, more women working outside the home and more single households.

Consumer demands are likely to continue to change into the future. By 2030, there may be more job sharing and more leisure time but less affluence. A lower proportion of the population will be working to support a higher proportion of older people in the population. There will be more single households and possibly greater health awareness.

Contamination due to (mis-)behaviour by food handlers

Many foodborne illnesses arise because of human error. As shown in Fig. 1.3 and Box 4.3, many outbreaks could be prevented by modifying human behaviour. Mistakes made by food handlers are most often due to the lack of training and education but carelessness and complacency also play a role.

Direct contamination by food handlers who are ill is also a major problem. Food service operations like restaurants, hotels, nursing homes, schools and hospitals are faced with the constant threat of food contamination by workers. Again, poor training and education are at the root of this problem but low wages and high staff turnover are also at fault. Hourly paid workers have little incentive to adopt good food-safety practices, such as staying at home when they are ill, as absence from work can lead to economic hardship.

Which foods are most often linked with illness?

Most foodborne outbreaks are associated with animal products such as meat and poultry, followed by other protein-rich foods such as seafood, milk and eggs. This is illustrated in Fig. 4.4. However, as we have seen in Fig. 4.1, there are likely to be

Table 4.5 Main reasons for outbreaks of foodborne illness and underlying causes

Main reasons for outbreaks of foodborne illness	Underlying causes
Poor temperature control during cooking, cooling and storage: • inadequate heating/undercooking (temperature too low and/or cooking time too short) • inadequate cooling, especially when large quantities prepared • storage at room temperature when chill-storage is indicated • inadequate reheating • inadequate thawing • improper warm holding Cross-contamination Infected food handlers Poor personal hygiene Poor cleaning regimes and contaminated equipment Preparation too far in advance	Food-handler behaviour: • lack of training and education • carelessness • complacency
Contaminated raw and processed food	On-farm and processing errors

many more cases of illness in the community that are never confirmed or linked with any particular food type. Therefore, we don't really know the exact proportions of cases associated with any single food type. It must not be assumed that foods other than meat and poultry are inherently safer.

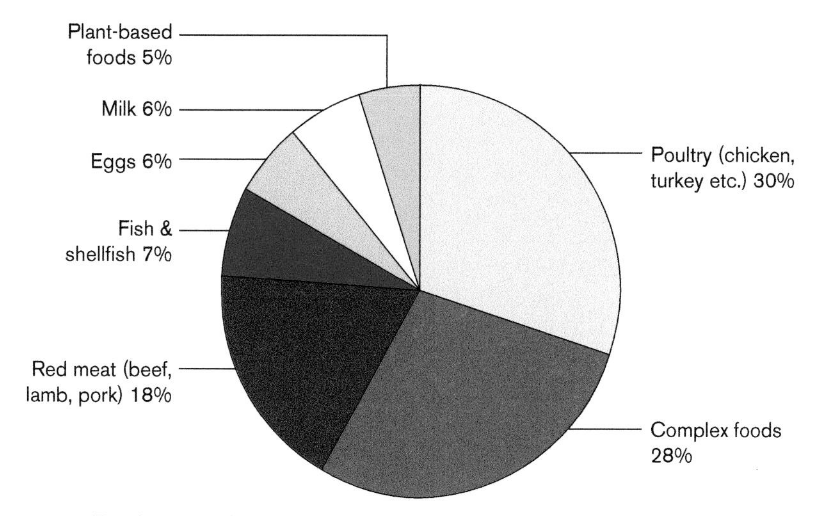

Figure 4.4 Foods most often identified as the source of illness in outbreaks. Complex foods are made up of several ingredients, often including meat. Plant-based foods include fruit, vegetables, salads and rice. Data from Adak *et al.* (2005); Batz *et al.* (2011).

Which organisms dominate the food-poisoning statistics?

Campylobacter and *Salmonella* cause hundreds of thousands of cases of foodborne illness every year and as such represent the 'world champions' of foodborne disease. *Listeria monocytogenes* and *Escherichia coli* O157:H7 cause far fewer cases of illness but are responsible for the highest number of deaths from foodborne illness. Although there are regional differences around the world, these four organisms dominate foodborne global statistics. In Chapters 5–7, we will explore all four, as well as several other important food pathogens, in more detail.

Food safety is a shared responsibility

The responsibility for ensuring the safety of our food is shared by many people from farmer through to home cook. Food handlers and consumers alike have a

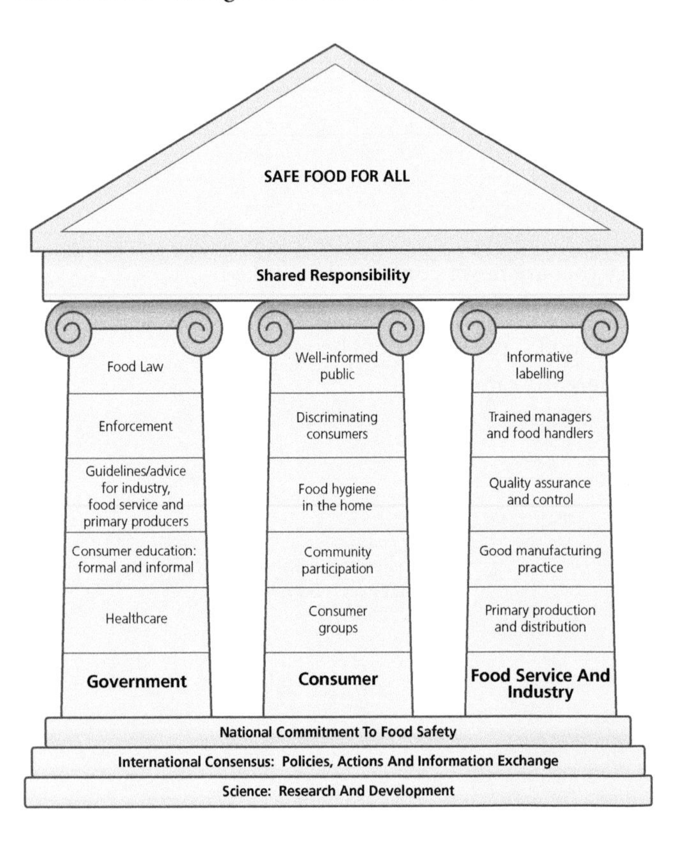

Figure 4.5 The Three Pillars of Food Safety. Government, consumers and industry/foodservice have a shared responsibility in assuring food safety for all. Source: World Health Organization (WHO).

role to play in maintaining a food supply that is as safe as possible. The concept of shared responsibility is illustrated in Fig. 4.5. The figure shows how good practices by governments, consumers and the food industry all underpin food safety. Without one of the three pillars, the edifice would collapse. For example, if the foodservice industry did not engage with food-safety practices, it would not be possible for governments and consumers alone to assure a safe food supply. It is only through a concerted effort by all that we can ensure that our foods are as safe as possible from plough to plate.

Chapter 4 Exercise

The UK Society for General Microbiology has devised an interactive online exercise based on a menu typically served in a cafeteria. Each dish on the menu is linked with microbes, some good, some bad and some ugly! It's fun to do and well worth a try, especially if you are new to food microbiology. Go to:
http://resources. schoolscience. co. uk/SGM/sgmfoods0.html

Chapter 4 Quiz

1 The number of foodborne cases of illness occurring globally is unacceptably high. Name five possible reasons for this.
2 Name five groups of people who are more likely to get sick and whose illness is likely to be more severe than in a healthy adult male.
3 Which four foodborne microbes are most often responsible for causing disease?
4 Name three food groups most often responsible for outbreaks of foodborne disease.
5 Food safety is a shared responsibility. Name the three main factors that must be in place to underpin food safety for all.

References and further reading

Adak, GK, Meakins, SM, Yip, H, Lopman, BA and O'Brien, SJ (2005). Disease risks from foods, England and Wales, 1996–2000. *Emerging Infectious Diseases* **11 (3)**: 365–72 (available from: **http://www. cdc. gov/ncidod/EID/ vol11no03/04-0191.htm**).

Batz, MB, Hoffmann, S and Morris, JG (2011). *Ranking the risks: The 10 pathogen-food combinations with the greatest burden on public health*. Emerging Pathogens Institute, University of Florida. Report and policy brief (available from: **http://epi. ufl. edu**).

Buckley, M and Reid, A (2010). *Global food safety: Keeping food safe from farm to table*. Report prepared on behalf of the American Academy of Microbiology (available from: **http://academy. asm. org**).

European Centre for Disease Prevention and Control (2010). *Annual epidemiological report on communicable diseases in Europe, 2010*. ECDC, Stockholm (available from: **http://www. ecdc. europa. eu/en/publications/ surveillance_reports/**).

Matheson, J (2010). The UK population: How does it compare? *Population Trends*, **142**: 9–32 (available from: **http:www. statistics. gov. uk/cci/article. asp?ID=2615**).

Scallan, E, Hoekstra RM, Angulo, FJ *et al.* (2011). Foodborne illness acquired in the United States. *Emerging Infectious Diseases*, **17 (1)**: 7–12 and 16–22 (available from: **http://www. cdc. gov/eid/content/17/1/7.htm**).

Scharff, RL (2010). *Health-related costs from foodborne illness in the United States* (available from: **http://www. producesafetyproject. org**).

Weblinks

For weblinks to international and national surveillance programmes and networks, see Box 4.2.

For all manner of information on global public health, visit the World Health Organization (WHO) website at:
http://www. who. int

The WHO food-safety pages are particularly relevant and provide the latest news, as well as detailed information on the work of international surveillance networks at:
http:www. who. int/foodsafety/en/

Factsheets on individual microbes and many other health issues are available and searchable at:
http://www. who. int/mediacentre/factsheets/

WHO Millennium Development Goals are available at:
http://www. who. int/mdg/goals/goal1/foodsafety/en/index. html

The website of the Food and Agriculture Organization of the United Nations provides a wealth of information on agricultural inputs and outputs, including food production at:
http://www. fao. org.

Pages concerned specifically with food safety and quality are at:
http://www. fao. org/ag/agn/agns

The United Nations makes regular projections of world population trends on a dedicated website at: **http://www. unpopulation. org**

The US Census Bureau provides a detailed database of worldwide population records at:
http://www. census. gov/ipc/www/idb/index. php

The European Food Safety Authority is at:
http://www. efsa. eu

The European Centre for Disease Prevention and Control (ECDC) is at:
http://ecdc. europa. eu

For all kinds of European statistics, visit the Eurostat site at:
http://epp. eurostat. ec. europa. eu/

For the latest statistics on foodborne disease in the UK, visit the UK Health Protection Agency at:
http://www. hpa. org. uk

and The Food Standards Agency at:
http://www. food. gov. uk

The US Centers for Disease Control and Prevention produces a wealth of information, including foodborne illness trends in the USA at:
http://www. cdc. gov/foodborneburden and

http://www. cdc. gov/FoodNet

http://www.edc.gov/outbreaknet/outbreaks.html

The US Department of Agriculture (USDA) includes the Food Safety Inspection Service at:
http://www. fsis. usda. gov

The *Bad Bug Book*, a handbook of foodborne pathogenic microorganisms (bacteria, viruses and parasites) and natural toxins provides basic facts about the most important foodborne microbes and poisons including characteristics, source, associated foods, infective dose, symptoms and outbreaks. The handbook is intended to bring together in one place information from the FDA, the CDC, the USDA Food Safety Inspection Service and the National Institutes of Health. It is available from:
http://www. fda. gov/Food/FoodSafety/FoodborneIllness/

Other useful websites

http://www. foodstandards. gov. au for the Food Standards Australia and New Zealand agency

http://www. anzfa. gov. au

http://www. ozfoodnet. gov. au for surveillance data in Australia

The Canadian Food Inspection Agency is at:
http://www. inspection. gc. ca

and Health Canada is at:
http://www. hc-sc. gc. ca

For further details on how foodborne outbreaks are investigated, the WHO book *Foodborne disease outbreaks: Guidelines for investigation and control* is available for downloading from:
http://www. who. int/foodsafety/publications/foodborne_disease/ fdbmanual/en/index. html

In the US, the CDC also provides a wealth of resources and an outbreak investigation toolkit, available for downloading from:
http://www. cdc. gov/outbreaknet/references_resources/

5

The reigning champions of food poisoning: *Campylobacter* and *Salmonella*

In this chapter, we examine *Campylobacter* and *Salmonella* bacteria together for two reasons. First, they are the two most frequently identified causes of food poisoning in the industrialized world. Second, many of the control measures available are equally effective against both bacteria. However, they also have some fundamental differences. In the following paragraphs, we compare and contrast these two important bacterial pathogens.

The size of the problem

Foodborne illness caused by *Campylobacter* has increased alarmingly since the 1970s. As shown in Fig. 5.1, the number of reported cases of campylobacteriosis (the illness caused by *Campylobacter*) per year in England and Wales is continuing to rise, despite a dip in the early 2000s. Trends in Europe have also been upward, with nearly 200 000 cases notified in 2009 alone. As the illness caused by *Campylobacter* is largely sporadic and unreported, the actual number of cases is

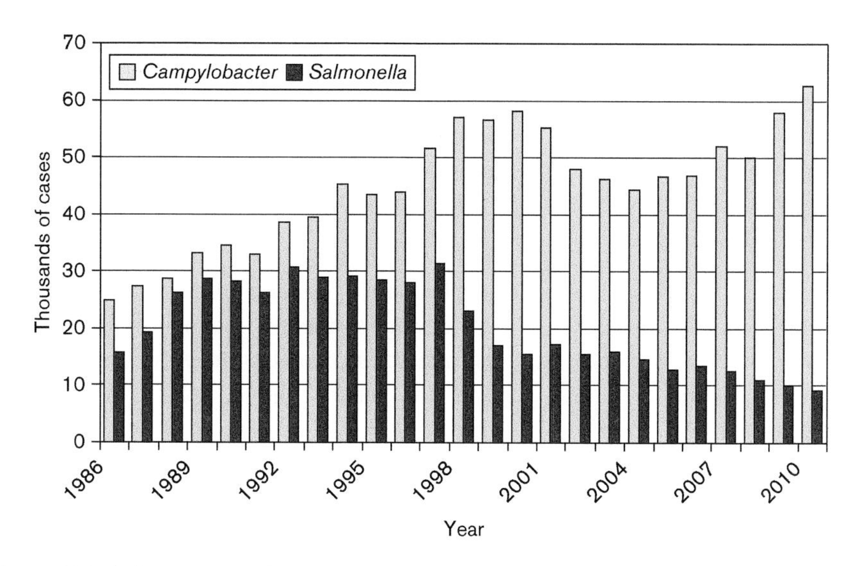

Figure 5.1 Laboratory-confirmed cases of illness caused by *Campylobacter* and *Salmonella* in England and Wales. Data from Health Protection Agency, UK (2011).

believed to be well over 1 million. In the USA, it has been estimated that up to 2 million cases per year may be attributable to *Campylobacter*. Similar upward trends have also been observed in other developed countries.

Despite more than three decades of intensive scientific research into *Campylobacter*, the organism remains somewhat of a mystery. This microbe is famously fussy: it needs micro-aerobic conditions (less oxygen than is normally present in air) to grow at its best, it does not grow at all at room temperature, requiring a minimum of 32°C, and it is sensitive to drying, heat and salt. So how could an organism that is considered by some microbiologists as 'a bit of a wimp' become such a successful foodborne pathogen? We don't know the answer yet but the low infective dose, the ability to stick to surfaces and the lack of an effective vaccine have all been suggested as contributing factors.

Campylobacter has overtaken *Salmonella* as the number one cause of human gastroenteritis in the developed world. But *Salmonella* is still responsible for causing the biggest number of outbreaks, large and small, from commercially produced and home-cooked foods, in large institutions and individual households, and often during special events such as weddings and barbeques. Some examples of very large foodborne outbreaks caused by *Salmonella* are shown in Table 4.4 and the story of Typhoid Mary is told in Box 5.1. Although the overall numbers of cases

Box 5.1 Microbiology Hall of Fame: Typhoid Mary (1869–1938)

Mary Mallon, nicknamed 'Typhoid Mary', became infamous in the early twentieth century when she caused at least 10 outbreaks of typhoid fever, 53 cases of illness and three deaths in New York City. She was an excellent example of a healthy **carrier**, a person who harbours a pathogenic organism and infects others without showing any outward symptoms of disease.

Mary worked as a domestic cook for 10 years and caused 28 cases of typhoid fever before the link was made between her and the illness. She was arrested in 1906 and admitted to an isolation hospital where it was discovered that her stools contained very large numbers of typhoid bacteria. She was eventually released after promising not to cook for others or serve food to anyone. Having no other obvious means of earning a living, Mary changed her surname and went back to work as a cook. For the next 5 years she infected at least as many people again. Eventually, she was tracked down and held in prison where she died in 1938.

In the past, typhoid fever killed thousands of people, mainly through water contaminated with sewage. Although less common in industrialized countries today, *Salmonella typhi*, the cause of typhoid fever, is still a major killer in the developing world. Most of the *Salmonella* outbreaks in the developed world today are caused by non-typhoidal strains.

of salmonellosis reported to public health authorities has been decreasing steadily in many developed countries (Fig. 5.1 and Table 4.2), *Salmonella* outbreaks still feature regularly in news headlines.

Overall, the levels of illness caused by *Campylobacter* and *Salmonella* are unacceptably high. Most, if not all, illnesses caused by these two bacteria could and should be preventable.

Tackling the problem at source: *Campylobacter* and *Salmonella* on the farm

Campylobacter and *Salmonella* co-exist with many wild animals and birds as well as pets and domestic animals used for food (see Microbial CVs). Animals contaminate the soil with their droppings and so it is not surprising that the bacteria have been isolated from root vegetables such as potatoes, sweet potatoes and carrots, as well as green leafy crops such as cabbage, lettuce, spinach, parsley and basil. Other fresh produce such as peppers, spring onions, cucumbers, radishes and mushrooms may also harbour *Campylobacter* and *Salmonella*.

Campylobacter can survive for several weeks in water provided it is at a relatively cool 10°C. *Salmonella* is more resilient and can survive in soil for up to 2 years and on potatoes and carrots for up to 40 days. Wild animals, soil and contaminated water provide a continuous source of these bacteria that is recycled between them and passed on to domestic animals and food crops. Under these circumstances, preventing contamination of plants and animals intended for human consumption is difficult.

Campylobacter and *Salmonella* thrive in the gut of chickens whose body temperature is 41–42°C. The organisms can multiply and reach very high numbers but the birds don't get sick. Young chicks can become colonized by the two organisms within 2 weeks of hatching. Once the microbes spread to an entire flock, the environment where the flock is housed quickly becomes contaminated too. For example, *Campylobacter* has been isolated from puddles outside sheds and even in air up to 30 m downwind from contaminated hen houses. The hands, footwear and cars of personnel working on chicken farms are also often contaminated by the two organisms. Contaminated broilers (chickens intended for meat production) then pass on the organism to other birds via transport crates and equipment used in slaughter houses.

Contamination of broiler houses and flocks can be kept in check by stringent biosecurity measures to avoid the horizontal spread of *Campylobacter* and *Salmonella* from the environment to poultry. In some countries such as New Zealand, a range of poultry industry interventions introduced in 2006 has led to remarkable reductions in the number of cases of illness reported to public health

Microbial CV *Campylobacter*

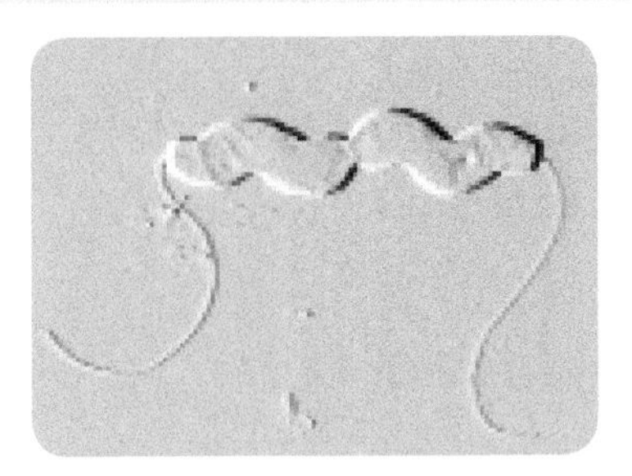

Atomic force micrograph of two *Campylobacter* cells head-to-head.

Photo credit: UK Institute of Food Research.

Home address: Intestines of wild and domestic birds, cattle, pigs, sheep, pets (dogs and cats), rodents (rats and mice), insects (especially flies).

Family background: A total of 16 species in the *Campylobacter* genus but *Campylobacter jejuni* and *C. coli* most important in relation to human health. *C. lari* and *C. upsaliensis* also occasionally cause illness.

Appearance: Gram negative, spiral-shaped rods, usually 0.2–0.5 µm wide and 0.5–5 µm long. Flagella (tails) propel the cell rapidly in a corkscrew-like manner.

Life skills: Ideal growth temperature 42°C. No growth below 30°C. Preferred atmosphere micro-aerobic where the normal oxygen content of air has been reduced from 21 per cent to 7 per cent. Sensitive to dry, salty or acidic conditions. Very sensitive to heat.

Unusual qualities: No growth in foods, only in living chickens, which do not become ill. Unlike *Salmonella*, cases tend to be sporadic with relatively few outbreaks.

Mode of transport to human victim

- Bird droppings, animal faeces, soil.
- Raw or undercooked poultry (chicken, including liver; duck, turkey, goose).
- Meat, unpasteurized milk, untreated water.

Disease-causing skills: Excellent. It takes just 500 cells to give you severe (and often bloody) diarrhoea, abdominal cramps, nausea and fever. If you're weak, as few as 100 cells will do the job nicely. 'Flu'-like symptoms start within 2–11 days of eating the affected food. Illness lasts up to 3 weeks. Live organisms may be passed in faeces for up to 12 weeks. Up to 10 per cent of patients develop complications such as stiffness, breathlessness, visual disturbances and headaches. Guillain-Barré syndrome, an autoimmune disease causing paralysis, may follow. Particularly nasty with children under the age of 4 years and the elderly. Number of cases of illness double in the summer months.

Achievements: Reigning champion of food poisoning, causing several tens of thousands of cases of illness in many industrialized countries every year. Has overtaken *Salmonella* in the food-poisoning race.

Microbial CV *Salmonella*

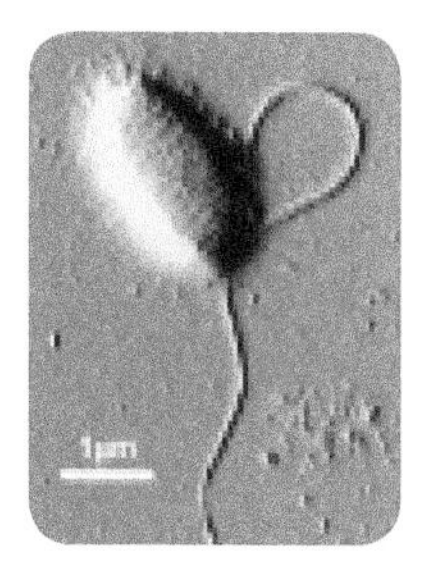

Atomic force micrograph of *Salmonella*.

Photo credit: Roy Bongaerts and Patrick Gunning, Institute of Food Research, UK.

Home address: Intestines of wild and domestic animals and birds (chickens, ducks and turkey), exotic pets (snakes, turtles, iguanas), frogs, rodents (rats and mice), beetles, cockroaches, worms, houseflies, tropical fish.

Family background: Over 2400 known species and strains in *Salmonella* genus. Most numerous species is *Salmonella enterica*.

Appearance: Gram negative, straight rods, 0.7–1.5 µm wide and 2–5 µm long. Flagella (tails) help with rapid movement.

Life skills: More resilient than *Campylobacter*. Can grow at room temperature but ideal is 37°C, with or without air. Cannot grow below 5°C or above 46°C. Sensitive to acids and easily killed by heat.

Unusual qualities: Can infect the hen's egg before the shell is formed and without making the hen ill. Good at surviving in fatty and dried foods.

Mode of transport to human victim

- Bird droppings, animal faeces, manure, soil.
- Raw or undercooked chicken and eggs.
- Meat, unpasteurized milk.
- Fatty foods such as chocolate, peanut butter, salami, cheddar cheese, mayonnaise.
- Dry foods such as spray-dried milk and ground spices (paprika, pepper, coriander).
- Bean and alfalfa sprouts, fresh fruit such as melons and tomatoes, salad vegetables such as peppers, rocket and lettuce, herbs such as basil.

Disease-causing skills: Excellent. It takes just 1000 cells to give you a bout of diarrhoea, abdominal cramps, vomiting and fever within 12–72 hours of eating the affected food. If the food is fatty, such as cheddar cheese, 500 cells are enough to cause illness and in chocolate even 50 cells may be enough. Illness lasts 2–7 days. Symptoms more severe in young children and the elderly. Number of cases triples in Europe during the summer months.

Achievements: Overtaken by *Campylobacter* in the numbers stakes, but still famous because of ability to cause many large outbreaks. Responsible for bringing multinational chocolate makers and peanut butter processors to their knees. Also very effective on the smaller scale, from children's petting farms to individual households.

authorities in the subsequent 2 years. One of the key measures introduced was the setting of mandatory (required by law) targets for the maximum number of *Campylobacter* allowed on poultry carcasses at the end of the slaughtering process. However, this option works only where birds are kept in closed housing conditions. With free-range birds and on cattle farms, prevention of contamination is difficult to achieve consistently. Good animal husbandry and agricultural practices can help to reduce the level of contamination of primary foodstuffs but they can never eliminate the presence of the organisms completely. *Campylobacter*- or *Salmonella*-free raw foods are impossible to guarantee at source.

The prevention of contamination with *Campylobacter* and *Salmonella* requires control measures at all stages of the food chain, from farm to fork. This includes interventions at the agricultural production stage through slaughtering, processing, manufacturing and finally preparation of foods in commercial and domestic settings.

Salmonella in eggs

Unlike *Campylobacter*, *Salmonella* can also be found in eggs. The organism can penetrate the egg sac inside the reproductive canal of the hen before the shell is formed. Once the egg is laid, *Salmonella* can also manoeuvre its way from droppings through the porous shell into a previously clean egg.

In the late 1980s, contamination of UK eggs with *Salmonella* was so widespread that it threatened the egg production industry and ultimately led to the resignation of a Health Minister. Since then, the incidence of *Salmonella* in eggs has been reduced dramatically by introducing a raft of on-farm and process control measures, embodied in the 'Lion Quality' Code of Practice (available from: http://www.lioneggs.co.uk). The most important of these measures was a mass vaccination programme for hens against *Salmonella*. In addition, each egg was labelled with a 'best before' date giving it a shelf-life of 21 days after laying. Storage temperatures below 20°C were also prescribed. Caterers were advised to use pasteurized egg in lightly cooked or uncooked dishes. A mass education campaign aimed at consumers in vulnerable groups recommended that raw eggs should be avoided when preparing dishes for the elderly, young children or the immuno-compromised. By 2007, a survey of over 1500 British eggs collected from catering premises showed that less than 1 per cent contained *Salmonella*.

So are eggs off the hook in terms of causing salmonellosis? Not for a minute! In the 2007 UK survey mentioned above, up to 7 per cent of imported eggs were contaminated with *Salmonella*. Furthermore, outbreaks of the illness continue to be linked with eggs, whether produced in the UK or other countries. For example, in 2011, *Salmonella* from eggs traced to a single shed on a farm in Spain sickened 262 people in the UK.

In 2010, *Salmonella* provoked a major US outbreak linked with eggs. An increase of nearly 2000 cases of salmonellosis over and above normal levels was detected by public health authorities. There were no deaths but the multistate outbreak caused illness at numerous restaurants and catered events. The outbreak was traced to eggs supplied by a single producer in Iowa. *Salmonella* was isolated from manure, walkways, equipment and feed mills in and around the farms. The egg firm conducted a voluntary recall of over 500 million eggs.

There is a clear need for continued vigilance when handling eggs. Poor handling practices by foodservice staff can increase the risk of infection by *Salmonella* in eggs. A 2007 UK study showed that more than half of the catering premises surveyed did not store their eggs under refrigerated conditions. One fifth of the eggs were still in use after their 'best before' dates had expired indicating poor stock rotation. Other surveys have revealed that raw eggs were shelled, pooled and stored at room temperature for up to 6 hours in about 25 per cent of US and 37 per cent of UK restaurants.

Survival of *Campylobacter* in food and water

Although *Campylobacter* cannot grow at room temperature, this is no handicap for the organism as it is quite capable of surviving in food and water and causing illness in very low numbers. As few as 100 cells can cause campylobacteriosis in young children, the elderly and other vulnerable people (for a full list of vulnerable people, see Chapter 4, p. 54).

Despite being relatively sensitive to oxygen, drying, acids and salt, *Campylobacter* can survive in raw chicken and beef at 20°C for a whole week. Chilling or freezing these foods reduces the numbers of *Campylobacter* present initially but these treatments do not eliminate the organism altogether. On the contrary, chilling and freezing can extend the survival time of *Campylobacter*. As shown in Table 5.1, reducing the storage temperature of raw chicken and cooked minced beef from 10°C to 2°C doubles the survival time of *Campylobacter*. The organism has even been isolated from raw beef and chicken after freezing for several months. However, the acidity of yogurt kills the organism in minutes, even at chill temperatures.

Unlike *Campylobacter*, *Salmonella* can not only survive but can also grow and multiply at room temperature, especially if it finds itself in a protein-rich food such as chicken or egg. Salmonella has been detected in egg droplets dried on surfaces more than 3 months after deposition. Like *Campylobacter*, *Salmonella* is generally sensitive to acids but can survive low-acid apple juice for more than 30 days.

Table 5.1 Survival of *Campylobacter* in a range of foods stored at different temperatures. Data from Bell and Kyriakides (2009).

Storage temperature (°C)	Food or water	Survival time
25	Water, non-carbonated mineral	Undetectable after 5 days
10	Chicken breast, raw	13 days
10	Beef, minced and cooked	23 days
4	Water, tap	More than 28 days
4	Raw milk	25 days
4	Yogurt	Less than 20 minutes
2	Chicken breast, raw	24 days
2	Beef, minced and cooked	49 days
−18	Beef strips, raw	3 months
−20	Chicken carcasses	4 months

The problem with chicken

Surveys have shown that in the UK, Germany and the USA, around 70 per cent of fresh retail chicken is contaminated with *Campylobacter.* In 2010, the European Food Safety Authority (EFSA) estimated that 80 per cent of chicken carcasses on the European Union market were contaminated with *Campylobacter.* In a New Zealand study, over 90 per cent of raw chicken portions and whole chickens tested positive for *Campylobacter.* The incidence is lower (up to 25 per cent) in raw retail beef, pork and lamb but still high enough to cause concern. The organism has also been isolated from nearly 10 per cent of samples from raw milk and cheeses made from unpasteurized milk.

Raw poultry meat is the food source most often responsible for cases of campylobacteriosis. The link between poultry and infection with *Campylobacter* was demonstrated particularly clearly in the late 1990s when chemical contamination with dioxin forced the authorities in Belgium to withdraw all poultry from the market for 4 weeks. Not only was the dioxin problem resolved but illnesses from *Campylobacter* dropped by a dramatic 40 per cent during the same time period. But given the popularity, excellent nutritional value and low price of chicken, it is unlikely that a complete ban on its sale and availability would be a realistic option for solving the problem of *Campylobacter* and *Salmonella.*

In countries such as the USA and New Zealand, chicken carcasses are sometimes washed with chlorinated or acidic water after slaughter. These treatments are effective up to a point: they reduce the level of contamination with *Campylobacter* and *Salmonella* but they do not eliminate the organisms entirely. Furthermore, antibacterial treatments are not permitted in many countries, most notably in Europe. It is possible to eliminate all bacteria from chicken by irradiation but continuing consumer opposition to this technology makes it an unlikely solution to the chicken problem in the foreseeable future.

Survival of *Campylobacter* and *Salmonella* in the kitchen

Many outbreaks of foodborne illness are linked with more than one cause. In the case of *Campylobacter* and *Salmonella*, outbreaks are most often associated with

Box 5.2 *Salmonella*: more than one reason for outbreaks

Kebab house in London, UK
207 cases, 31 hospitalized
Food source: Chicken kebab
Salmonella was also isolated from 14 other food samples, three members of staff who had been unwell but continued to work, and a wiping cloth
Reasons for outbreak: Contaminated raw material (chicken), inadequate heating (kebab), cross-contamination through poor hygienic practices, poor training of staff

Vegetarian restaurant in Stockholm, Sweden
115 cases, 13 hospitalized
Food source: Mung beans soaked overnight at room temperature to soften
Reasons for outbreak: Contaminated raw material (beans imported from Canada), inappropriate processing and storage temperature

Nursery school in UK
147 cases, mainly young children
Food source: Raw eggs
Salmonella was also isolated from 'clean' mixing bowls and chopping boards
Reasons for outbreak: Contaminated raw material (eggs), vulnerable group, cross-contamination through poor hygienic practices, inadequate cleaning, poor training of staff

Hotel restaurant in northern England
15 cases, three elderly patients hospitalized, one person died
Food source: Tiramisu made with raw shell eggs
Reasons for outbreak: Contaminated raw material (despite buying eggs from *Salmonella*-vaccinated sources only), vulnerable group

Box 5.3 *Campylobacter*: more than one reason for outbreaks

Restaurant in Oklahoma, USA
14 cases, 2 hospitalized
Food sources: Lettuce and lasagne
Reasons for outbreak: Kitchen surfaces contaminated from raw chicken prepared earlier in the day, inadequate cleaning of chopping boards and utensils, poor hand hygiene, chef's towel around waist, chef received no training in food hygiene

Hawaiian theme restaurant, UK
12 cases
Food source: Stir-fried chicken in 'Sizzling Wok Special'
Reasons for outbreak: Contaminated raw material (chicken pieces), variable thickness of chicken strips, inadequate cooking during peak times, no hygiene training of food handlers

School in Madrid, Spain
81 cases, all school children, 31 visited doctor
Food sources: Custard
Reasons for outbreak: Milk used to make custard was cross-contaminated from raw chicken used to make paella on day before meal was served, custard stored at room temperature, poor hygienic practices in kitchen, inadequate food-safety training

Wedding reception at luxury hotel in northern England
24 cases, one hospitalized
Food sources: Chicken liver parfait
Reasons for outbreak: Contaminated raw material (chicken livers), parfait heated in bain-marie to core temperature of 65°C but not held at this temperature for any length of time before cooling

two main factors: undercooking and cross-contamination. Some examples of these are shown in Boxes 5.2 and 5.3.

Raw poultry is one of the most important sources of contamination in a kitchen, whether commercial or domestic. All raw poultry products must be treated as contaminated, irrespective of the storage conditions. *Campylobacter* has been detected on up to 40 per cent of external surfaces of packaging used to wrap whole chicken in UK supermarkets. Therefore, even the packaging that the poultry arrives in should be treated as contaminated.

Campylobacter and *Salmonella* are transferred readily from chicken to hands, chopping boards, knives and sponges used for washing up. As shown in Table 5.2, *Campylobacter* was detected on nearly all hands, chopping boards and washing up cloths used by 20 food handlers after cutting up a raw chicken. Furthermore, about half of the food handlers had more than the minimum infective dose of

Campylobacter on their hands after preparing the chicken. In another study, *Campylobacter* was transferred from raw chicken to kitchen utensils and then to ready-to-eat food on about one third of occasions observed in a professional kitchen.

Table 5.2 Proportion of hands, chopping boards and dishcloths contaminated with *Campylobacter* during preparation of raw chicken. Data from Cogan *et al* (2002). J Appl Microbiol. **92**, 885–892.

	Percentage of samples contaminated		
Number of *Campylobacter* detected	**Hands**	**Chopping board**	**Dishcloth used for washing up**
At least one	85	80	85
Between 100 and 1000	50	55	45
More than 1000	20	45	40

Brand new polypropylene chopping boards are generally very smooth and have fewer niches and crevices to shelter bacteria than chopping boards made of wood. However, once used, *Campylobacter* and *Salmonella* can survive on both plastic and wooden boards for up to 2 hours at room temperature. The extent to which bacteria stick to chopping boards depends more on the scoring or the level of use that the board has received than on the material from which the board is made.

A common misconception among professional chefs and home cooks alike is that it is necessary to wash raw chicken or chicken portions prior to cooking. Washing chicken is not only completely ineffective in removing bacteria but it actually helps to spread *Salmonella* and *Campylobacter* on to work surfaces, utensils and other foods up to 1 m away from the water source. This is illustrated in Fig. 5.2. Washing chicken represents bad practice and should not be done.

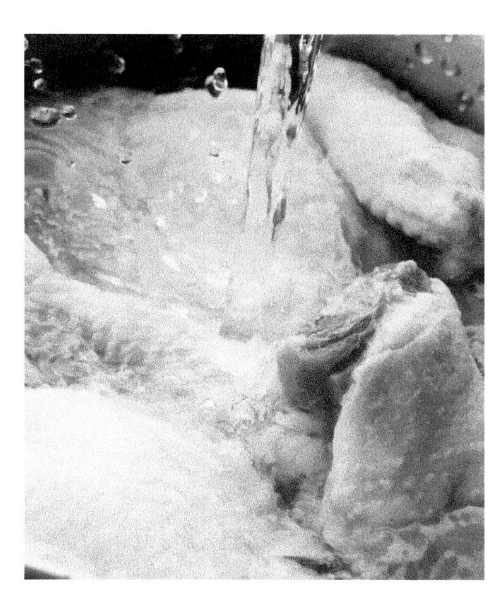

Figure 5.2 Washing chicken is a bad idea. Don't do it! Washing chicken creates droplets of water containing *Campylobacter* and *Salmonella*. These can land up to 1 m away from the chicken. Washing chicken spreads bacteria and can lead to illness (© Ian O'Leary/Dorling Kindersley/Getty Images).

Thorough washing up of all utensils and boards used in the kitchen helps to remove adhering microorganisms but their survival depends on the temperature of the water. The upper limit for growth of *Salmonella* and *Campylobacter* is about 46°C but the microbes can survive at this temperature for extended periods. For example, at 48°C (hand-hot water is about 45°C), *Salmonella* can survive for up to 30 minutes. If the temperature of the washing up water is raised to 52°C, *Salmonella* is killed off after 5 minutes. Since many automatic dishwashing machines have standard cycle temperatures of 60°C, it is clear that machine washing is preferable to hand washing for cleaning all utensils and chopping boards.

Poor cleaning practices, inadequate hand washing and undercooking all contribute significantly to the potential spread of infection by *Salmonella* and *Campylobacter* in both commercial and domestic kitchens. Measures used to control all these practices are covered in more detail in Chapter 8.

Chapter 5 Quiz

1. Name the two bacteria and the single food source most often responsible for food poisoning worldwide.
2. Outbreaks of foodborne illness are often caused by more than one cause. Name the two factors most often associated with *Salmonella* poisoning.
3. What is the preferred method of washing up after preparing raw chicken and why?
4. Which pair of foods must always be kept separate to avoid cross-contamination? (Select one pair only)
   - Raw potatoes and raw stewing steak.
   - Cooked chicken and a dressed, mixed-leaf salad.
   - Raw chicken portions and fresh tomato salad.
   - Raw, washed spring onions and cooked roast beef.
5. Which of the following foods served at a buffet is most likely to cause food poisoning? (Select one only)
   - Tuna and sweetcorn salad made with bottled mayonnaise.
   - French bread.
   - Mixed green salad dressed with oil and vinegar.
   - Barbequed chicken wings.
   - Crisps and peanuts.

Chapter 5 Exercises

Exercise 1

If some people are carriers of pathogenic bacteria without showing obvious signs of illness, how can we prevent the spread of disease in a food preparation area?

Tip: Name some of the possible prevention measures. Discuss the pros and cons of each measure and how it could be implemented in large, medium and small food businesses.

Exercise 2

Should the use of raw eggs in lightly cooked or uncooked foods such as mayonnaise and mousses be banned by law? Discuss.

Tip: Consider the needs of consumers in general as well as those in vulnerable groups. Compare and contrast the use of raw eggs in the large food manufacturing sector, foodservice establishments (restaurants, work canteens, nurseries, schools, prisons, hospitals, old people's homes) and the home.

Further reading

Bell, C and Kyriakides, A (2002). *Salmonella: A practical approach to the organism and its control in foods.* Wiley-Blackwell, Chichester, UK.

Bell, C and Kyriakides, A (2009). *Campylobacter: A practical approach to the organism and its control in foods.* Wiley-Blackwell, Chichester, UK.

Sears, A, Baker, MG, Wilson, N *et al.* (2011). Marked campylobacteriosis decline after interventions aimed at poultry, New Zealand. *Emerging Infectious Diseases*, **17 (6)**, 1007–15 (available online from: **http:www. cdc. gov/eid**).

Weblinks

The 'Lion Quality' Code of Practice for eggs is available from: **http://www. lioneggs. co. uk.**

Advice for caterers about safe handling of eggs can be found on: **http://www. food. gov. uk/news/newsarchive/2009/oct/eggssafe and**

http://www. food. gov. uk/foodindustry/caterers/eggs/

The EFSA has issued advice on reduction of *Campylobacter* in chicken. The full article 'Scientific opinion on *Campylobacter* in broiler meat production: control options and performance objectives and/or targets at different stages of the food chain' was published online in 2011 and is available from: **http://www. efsa. europa. eu/en/efsajournal/pub/2105.htm**

6

Less common but more deadly: *E. coli* and *Listeria*

In this chapter we discuss two microbes, the verocytotoxin-producing *Escherichia coli* (or VTEC for short) and *Listeria monocytogenes*. Compared with *Salmonella* and *Campylobacter*, these two pathogens cause less than one tenth the number of cases of illness but when they do strike, they are much more likely to kill the patient. Fatalities are particularly high in the elderly and the very young.

The problem with VTEC

Most strains of *E. coli* are harmless and live in the lower intestinal tract of healthy animals and humans. *E. coli* are relatively easy to detect in the laboratory and so are often used as **indicator organisms**. The presence of *E. coli* in a food or water indicates that faecal contamination has occurred and poor hygiene has been practised.

E. coli was discovered in 1885 by Dr Theodor Escherich and has since been studied extensively by researchers wishing to understand the basic principles of microbial biology. One of the strains, *E. coli* K-12, is very easy to grow in the laboratory and is considered so safe to handle that it is often used to teach microbiology in school laboratories. However, the early 1980s saw the emergence of a new pathogenic strain of *E. coli* with the ability to kill people. As a result, VTEC is often referred to as an **emerging pathogen**.

The different strains of *E. coli* are distinguished by the chemical composition of their cell surface. These differences can be measured using **antibodies** as reagents. Antibodies are very specific and will react only with molecules (**antigens**) with specific structures. These reactions have been developed into immunological test kits that allow classification of the different strains into **serotypes**. There are more than 170 serotypes in *E. coli* based on the O antigen (corresponding to the sugars on the outer membrane of the cell), over 100 based on the K antigen (cell capsule) and over 50 based on the H antigen (flagella). One of the most common pathogenic strains of *E. coli* is referred to as *E. coli* O157:H7, meaning that it has the O antigen 157 and the H antigen 7.

There are other strains of *E. coli* that also produce deadly toxins and these are sometimes referred to as shigatoxin producing *E. coli* or STEC, or enterohaemorrhagic *E. coli* or EHEC. In this chapter and throughout this book, we refer to all toxin-producing *E. coli* collectively as **verocytotoxin**-producing *Escherichia coli* or VTEC. The name 'verocytotoxin' comes from the method used in the laboratory to detect its presence. The method relies on culturing 'vero' cells originating from African green monkey kidneys in laboratory dishes.

As shown in the Microbial CV for VTEC, the pathogenic strains have a very low infective dose and are particularly dangerous for people aged over 65 years or under 5 years. In about 10 per cent of the cases, the initial enteric (gut-associated) symptoms (bloody diarrhoea and abdominal pain) are followed by haemolytic uraemic syndrome (HUS), a serious illness of the kidneys. Mortality is high for patients who develop the more serious symptoms.

Figure 6.1 shows that the number of cases of VTEC in the UK increased alarmingly in the 1990s. Of the 995 cases reported in 2000, 377 were hospitalized and 22 died. After a dip in the early 2000s, numbers started rising again, reaching an average of 800–1000 cases per year. The upward trend in the 1990s followed by more stable but high figures in the 2000s is reflected in Europe with more than 5000 cases reported in 2005 alone. In the USA, it is estimated that about 75 000 cases of VTEC occur annually.

A very close relative of *E. coli*, *Shigella*, causes hundreds of millions of cases of bacterial dysentery (bloody diarrhoea) worldwide and a million deaths every year. However, 99 per cent of the infections occur in developing countries. The illness is usually associated with contaminated water supplies and poor sanitary facilities. Person-to-person transmission is also common and 60 per cent of all deaths from

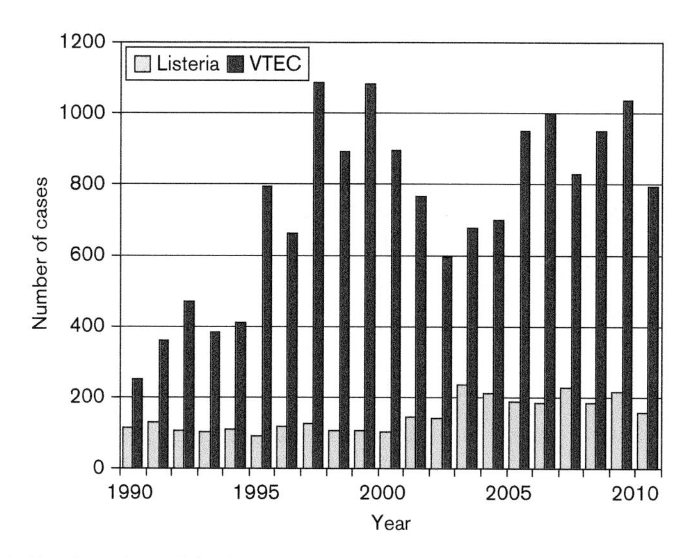

Figure 6.1 Number of confirmed cases of illness caused by verotoxigenic *Esherichia coli* (VTEC) and *Listeria monocytogenes* in England and Wales. Data from Health Protection Agency (HPA), UK (2011).

Microbial CV — Verocytotoxin-producing *Escherichia coli* (VTEC)

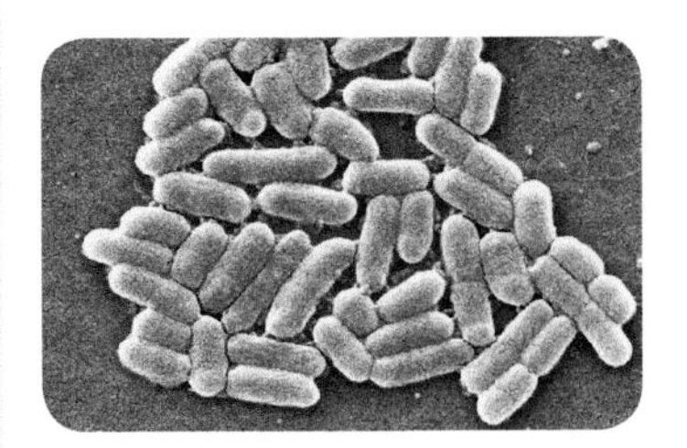

Verocytotoxin-producing *Escherichia coli*, Scanning Electron Micrograph, magnification 6836X.

Photo credit: CDC.

Main address: Intestines of healthy cattle.

Other addresses: Sheep, goats, water buffalo, rabbits and rodents; wild birds; slugs, worms, beetles, houseflies, fruitflies.

Family background: More than 320 types of *Escherichia coli*, distinguished mainly by the chemical composition of their cell surface. Most strains are harmless but a few like *E. coli* 0157:H7 and 0104:H4 can kill people.

Appearance: Gram negative, straight rods, about 0.5 μm wide and 2 μm long. Flagella (tails) help the organism to move around.

Life skills: Ideal growth temperature is 37°C but grows happily at 25°C and more slowly at lower temperatures. Can grow with or without oxygen. Sensitive to salt but relatively tolerant of acids and dry conditions. Like *Salmonella*, *Campylobacter* and *Listeria*, VTEC is very sensitive to heat. Can spread from person to person, or from animal to person (as on children's petting farms) as well as *via* food and water.

Unusual qualities: Pathogenic strains produce potent toxins (poisons) with severe consequences for the kidney, blood and the central nervous system. *E. coli* 0157:H7 is much more tolerant to acidic conditions than its non-pathogenic cousins.

Mode of transport to human victim:

- Animal faeces, soil, manure, sewage, untreated water
- Beef products including those produced organically e.g. undercooked burgers, steak tartare, raw milk, poorly prepared fermented sausages
- Green leafy vegetables such as spinach, lettuce and cabbage; herbs such as coriander; celery; sprouts from alfalfa, cress, fenugreek, mung beans and radish
- Apples, unpasteurised apple juice, mayonnaise

Disease-causing skills: Excellent. It takes just 10 to 100 cells to give you bloody diarrhoea and abdominal pain for up to 2 weeks. Symptoms start within 3 to 4 days of eating the contaminated food. Around 10% of cases develop Haemolytic Uraemic Syndrome (HUS), an illness of the kidneys. Kidney failure and death can follow, especially in the elderly and children under the age of 5. The number of cases of illness is highest in the late summer months.

Achievements: Relatively rare by comparison with *Campylobacter* or *Salmonella* but much more deadly.

shigellosis occur in children under the age of 5 years. In developed countries, foodborne outbreaks caused by *Shigella* are relatively rare.

VTEC outbreaks

Illness caused by VTEC is largely sporadic but several high-profile outbreaks have occurred and some examples of these are given in Box 6.1. Two large outbreaks that occurred in the UK are discussed in more detail below.

Lessons not learned from VTEC outbreaks in the UK

> 'That men do not learn very much from the lessons of history is the most important of all the lessons that history has to teach'
>
> *Aldous Huxley, 1959*

The largest VTEC outbreak in the UK occurred in Scotland in 1996. More than 500 people were made ill and 21 died. The majority of the people with serious

Box 6.1 VTEC:Examples of outbreaks

Fast food restaurant chain, USA, 1992/3
732 cases, 195 hospitalizations, 55 cases of Haemolytic Uraemic Syndrome (HUS), four deaths
Food source:Beefburgers
Reasons for outbreak:Contaminated ground beef used to make burgers, inadequate cooking

School lunches, Japan, 1996
9578 cases, mostly schoolchildren, 11 deaths
Food source:Radish sprouts
Reasons for outbreak:Contaminated seeds used by single supplier to produce radish sprouts

Multiple outlets, USA, 2006
205 cases, 103 hospitalizations, 31 cases of HUS, five deaths
Food source:Spinach
Reasons for outbreak:Raw spinach contaminated with agricultural run-off from cattle

Multiple restaurants and catering establishments, Germany and France, 2011
4178 cases, over 800 cases of HUS, 48 deaths
Food source:Sprouts made from fenugreek seeds imported from Egypt
Reason for outbreak:Contaminated fenugreek seeds used to grow sprouts for raw consumption

disease and all those who died were over the age of 60 years. The size and severity of the outbreak shocked the nation. A public inquiry chaired by Professor Hugh Pennington of the University of Aberdeen investigated the reasons for the outbreak and made 32 recommendations for improvement of food-safety practices. It was thought at the time that the lessons learned would prevent future problems.

The butcher responsible for the Scottish outbreak supplied both raw and cooked meat products to individuals and institutions. A church lunch attended by about 100 people, a birthday party held in a pub and meals taken at a nursing home were all involved in the outbreak. Investigations revealed that VTEC was present in the gravy and on the faulty boiler used to cook the steak for the church lunch, on the cooked ham supplied for the birthday party and on several joints of roast beef, pork and ham sold to individuals. The outbreak strain was found all over the butcher's premises, including a vacuum packing machine and on raw beef sirloin, beef sausage, stewing steak wrapped in plastic and legs of pork.

The Pennington inquiry identified several shortcomings with the procedures used by the butcher, the most important of which was the failure to prevent cross-contamination. In addition, the temperature reached by the meat products during cooking was too low to kill VTEC. Once cooked, the products were not cooled quickly enough, refrigeration was inadequate and there was evidence of poor cleaning practices. The proprietor had failed to implement a proper **Hazard Analysis Critical Control Point (HACCP)** plan (more on HACCP in Chapter 9). The butcher was prosecuted but there were also systemic failures in local government inspection procedures and enforcement of hygiene.

As a result of one of the recommendations, licensing of butchers' shops was introduced in the UK in May 2000. The licensing rules required butchers selling both unwrapped meat and ready-to-eat foods to be licensed on an annual basis by their local authority. To obtain a licence, butchers had to demonstrate a functioning HACCP plan, enhanced hygiene training of staff and good temperature control within their premises. The licensing scheme in England and Scotland was evaluated in 2002 and was shown to have improved hygiene standards in butchers' shops. However, the scheme was dropped at the end of 2005 because it was superseded by new European Union hygiene regulations that came into force in January 2006. These required all food businesses, including butchers' shops, to operate HACCP-based food safety procedures. The new European Union regulations were thought to provide an equivalent level of public health protection as the butchers' licensing scheme.

Some of the other recommendations of the Pennington group were also heeded. Central funding was made available to local authorities and several codes of practice and guidance notes were revised and improved. There was a sense of optimism that new measures would ensure that a similar outbreak would not recur.

But not all the lessons of the Scottish outbreak were learned. Nine years later, another large VTEC outbreak occurred in Wales, this time striking young children rather than the elderly. One boy, aged 5 years, died. Once again, Professor Pennington was asked to chair a new inquiry. The circumstances of the Welsh outbreak were uncannily similar to those leading to the Scottish one. Professor Pennington was not amused.

The Welsh outbreak was caused by cooked meats supplied to 44 schools by a catering butcher who also owned the abattoir (slaughterhouse) supplying his business. There were 157 cases (mainly schoolchildren) of which 31 were hospitalized and one 5-year-old boy died. The same strain of *E. coli* O157 isolated from patients was found in cooked meats recovered from several schools, in raw meat from the butcher's premises, and in cow faeces taken from a farm supplying cattle to the butcher. The business owner was charged with seven food hygiene offences, sentenced to 12 months in prison and banned from managing any food businesses in the future. As in the Scottish outbreak, the proprietor had repeatedly failed to separate raw and cooked meats, ensure that cleaning was carried out properly and implement a proper HACCP plan. As in Scotland, many of the systems intended to assure food safety including local government inspection procedures, the commissioning of school catering contracts and enforcement of abattoir hygiene were ineffective. The second Pennington inquiry produced 24 recommendations. The coroner at the inquest into the death of the 5-year-old boy who died recommended stronger enforcement of food hygiene laws.

It remains to be seen if there will be a third Pennington inquiry.

VTEC in fresh produce

A massive outbreak of bloody diarrhoea and HUS caused by a rare strain (O104:H4) of VTEC struck Europe in mid-2011. More than 4000 people were made ill, over 800 developed HUS and 48 people died. Unlike previous outbreaks in the UK and elsewhere affecting mainly the elderly or young children, most of the patients were women over the age of 20 years. The symptoms of illness were unusually severe and a high proportion of patients developed HUS. About half of the patients with HUS went on to develop neurological complications, including life-threatening seizures. The outbreak strain was eventually linked with raw sprouts made from fenugreek seeds imported from Egypt. Several national public health authorities issued revised guidance to consumers that sprouted seeds such as fenugreek and alfalfa as well as mung beans should not be eaten raw and should be thoroughly cooked until steaming hot throughout.

Tackling the VTEC problem

Healthy cattle are carriers of VTEC and shed large numbers of the microbe in their faeces. Some animals excrete very large numbers of VTEC and are known as super-shedders or **super-spreaders**. Like Typhoid Mary, who was a healthy human spreader of *Salmonella* (see Box 5.1), VTEC is spread by some animals more than others. Since high numbers may be present in faeces, VTEC transfers easily to carcasses during slaughter or to milk during milking. VTEC survives readily in soil, sawdust, walls and roof of animal housing for up to 10 months.

Although there are measures that can be taken on the farm to reduce the level of contamination with VTEC, the widespread nature of *E. coli* means that complete elimination of the microbe from raw agricultural products is impossible to guarantee. Therefore, it must be assumed that any raw beef ingredient or food crop produced with the aid of manure or irrigation water may be contaminated with *E. coli* at the point of delivery to the kitchen or food processor. Relevant Control Points (discussed in more detail in Chapter 8) must be in place to reduce the hazards during processing and to prevent recontamination of processed products.

The problem with *Listeria*

Listeria monocytogenes was first isolated and named in the 1920s but like VTEC, it was not recognized as a serious foodborne pathogen until the 1980s. Several notable outbreaks in the early 1980s alerted microbiologists, healthcare professionals and the general public to the growing problem of listeriosis. To this day, the number of cases occurring worldwide is relatively small (about 200 in the UK and 1500 each in Europe and the USA) by comparison with the hundreds of thousands of illnesses caused by *Salmonella* and *Campylobacter*. But with fatality rates as high as 40 per cent, listeriosis continues to be a major cause for concern (Table 6.1).

Table 6.1 Some examples of large listeriosis outbreaks. Data from Bell and Kyriakides (2005), Health Canada, UK Health Protection Agency (HPA) and US Centers for Disease Control (CDC)

Year	Source	Number of cases	Number of deaths	Mortality rate (per cent)	Location
1980–1981	Coleslaw	41	18	44	Canada
1983–1987	Vacherin Mont D'Or cheese	122	34	29	Switzerland
1985	Mexican-style cheese	142	48	34	California, USA
1987–1989	Pâté made by single Belgian manufacturer	366	63	17	UK
1992	Pork tongue in aspic	279	63	23	France
2008	Delicatessen meat	57	22	39	Canada
2011	Cantaloupe melons	146	30	21	USA

Microbial CV *Listeria monocytogenes*

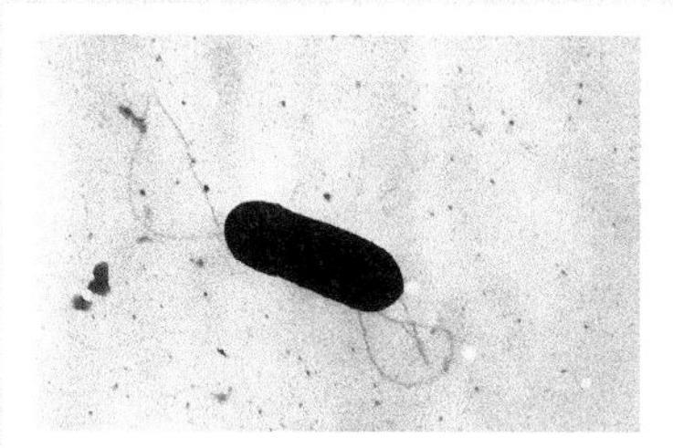

Listeria monocytogenes, Transmission Electron Micrograph, magnification 41,250X.

Photo credit: CDC.

Home address: Not fussy. Lives on and in plants, animals, soil, water, everywhere!

Family background: There are six species in the *Listeria* genus but *Listeria monocytogenes* is most often associated with human illness.

Appearance: Gram positive, short rods, about 0.9 µm long and 0.5 µm wide. Flagella (tails) enable the organism to move by "tumbling".

Life skills: Ideal growth temperature is 37°C but grows happily at temperatures well below those of most refrigerators. Can grow with or without oxygen. Relatively resistant to drying. Can grow in the presence of 10% salt and survive in as much as 25%. Like *Salmonella*, *Campylobacter* and VTEC, it is very sensitive to heat.

Unusual qualities: Unlike *Salmonella*, *Campylobacter* and VTEC, *Listeria* can grow at 0.5 to 3°C, making it a particular menace in the refrigerator.

Mode of transport to human victim:

- Unpasteurized milk, all cheeses made from unpasteurized milk, surface-ripened cheeses like brie and camembert, blue-veined cheeses like stilton, butter, ice cream
- Pâté and rillettes, pork tongue in aspic, all kinds of deli meats, sliced cooked turkey and chicken, bologna sausage, frankfurters
- Coleslaw salad, rice salad, pickled olives, cut melon, hummus dip
- Seafood including shrimps, smoked mussels, smoked salmon, cod's roe
- Chilled, ready-to-eat foods such as sandwiches

Disease-causing skills: Not so good with healthy, young adults but particularly accomplished at making older people and newborn babies ill. Can cross the placenta to infect unborn babies without making the mother ill. Patients with cancer, HIV/AIDS or organ transplants receiving immuno-suppressing drugs are also very vulnerable. Flu-like symptoms start 3 to 8 days after eating contaminated food but may take as long as 90 days to appear. Illness lasts several weeks, sometimes months. Complications are very serious: septicaemia (blood poisoning), meningitis (infection of tissues surrounding the brain), miscarriage, stillbirth. Cases peak in the summer months. Up to 5% of humans can be carriers without any signs of disease.

Achievements: Relatively rare by comparison with *Campylobacter* or *Salmonella* but much more deadly especially for unborn babies and people aged over 60.

In the 1980s, the group of people most affected by *Listeria* and subsequent complications (see Microbial CV for *Listeria*) were expectant mothers and their unborn and newborn babies. Babies often died from listeriosis. Following several national and successful public health campaigns advising pregnant women to avoid unpasteurized dairy products, surface-ripened and blue-veined cheeses, and pâté, the number of pregnancy-related cases of listeriosis decreased substantially in many countries. However, since 2001, the illness has been on the rise again in the UK and several European countries, including France, Germany, Spain, Belgium, Denmark and the Netherlands. This time, a different vulnerable group was affected: people over the age of 60 years.

More than half of all listeriosis cases are now occurring in people aged 60 years or more. In the UK, the rate of listeriosis in those over 60 years has increased threefold from 1990 to 2010 and is too large to be explained away by an ageing population or by improved diagnostics. Patients over 60 years are more likely to suffer from bacteraemia (presence of bacteria in blood) than meningitis (infection of tissues surrounding the brain). The older the patient, the more likely they are to die from the illness. Recent research also suggests that the group of vulnerable people may be somewhat wider than previously thought. In addition to patients on immuno-suppressing drugs (for treating cancer or preventing organ rejection after transplants), otherwise healthy people taking medication to suppress stomach acids and the burning sensation of acid reflux may also be at higher risk from infection by *Listeria*. Other conditions such as diabetes and heart disease also seem to predispose people to listeriosis.

Listeriosis is difficult to diagnose correctly as the incubation period can be as long as 3 months. The early symptoms are very much like those of influenza ('flu'). Laboratory tests to confirm the diagnosis might not be ordered until the patient becomes critically ill, leaving less time for treatment to take effect. The long incubation period also makes it difficult to make the link between the illness and a specific food.

Most cases of listeriosis are sporadic, although high-profile outbreaks still occur. The Canadian outbreak of 2008 is worthy of mention here, not least because it culminated in the death of 22 elderly people from listeriosis (Table 6.1). The average age of the people who died was 76 years. Almost 80 per cent of those who developed listeriosis lived in long-term residential care or were already in hospital for treatment of other diseases. The outbreak was traced to delicatessen meats supplied by a single producer. Like the Pennington inquiries into the two VTEC outbreaks in the UK, a high-level investigation into the reasons for the outbreak was commissioned by the Canadian Government. The Canadian Independent Investigator published a 181-page report on the findings and made 57 recommendations for improvement of food-safety practices. As is often the case in large outbreaks, there were multiple causes, including systemic weaknesses in the producing company and the public sector. For example, senior managers at the meat-processing plant were aware that *Listeria* was repeatedly detected in some of the productionlines for up to 1 year before the outbreak. The lines were sanitized using standard industry procedures but the head office of the company was not informed because local managers believed that the problem was under control. Furthermore, the company was producing large packages of delicatessen meats for sale to institutions and had reduced the levels of salt in the recipes in order to service clients on low-sodium diets. There were issues around the capacity and training of food-hygiene inspectors and the state of readiness of the various local, regional and national authorities to deal with an emergency. The national strategy for communicating with the public in the event of an outbreak was also found wanting. The investigation report concluded that the Canadian Government should make food safety a top priority.

Like the Pennington inquiries in the UK, many of the issues raised and even some of the recommendations made by the Canadian investigation, were not new. Until recommendations made in such reports are turned into actions, similar outbreaks are likely to recur.

A key difference between *Listeria* and many other pathogenic bacteria is its ability to grow at refrigeration temperatures. Consequently, foods associated with *Listeria* are usually ready-to-eat, refrigerated products with extended shelf-lives. In particular, foods that have not been heated (such as salads and sandwiches) or foods that may have been contaminated after cooking (e.g. during slicing of delicatessen meats) and then stored under chill conditions before eating, are considered high risk with respect to *Listeria monocytogenes*. Smoked fish and seafood prepared using cold-smoking processes at 30°C are also risky. In a UK survey of several thousand samples of cold-smoked salmon, nearly one fifth were found to contain *Listeria*. For a more complete list of foods affected, see Microbial CV for *Listeria*.

It is not clear if the changes in the epidemiology and clinical symptoms of listeriosis are due to changes in the **virulence** (ability to cause disease) of the organism, susceptibility of those over 60 years to the microbe, dietary behaviour or changes in food-production processes. More evidence is needed to pinpoint the exact cause of the changes. Meanwhile, many food manufacturers are making the presence of unpasteurized milk in products such as cheese more obvious by explicit labelling, allowing the consumer to make a better-informed choice during purchase.

Public health authorities in many countries are advising people over 60 years, as well as other vulnerable groups, about the life-threatening nature of *Listeria* and how to take simple steps to avoid being poisoned by the organism. For example, in 2009, the Food Standards Agency in the UK made *Listeria* the focus of its Food Safety Week, an event that takes place every year in June. Older people were advised to take care with chilled foods by ensuring that their refrigerators do not exceed 5°C and discarding foods that are past their **'use by' dates** (see Chapter 8, p. 136 for definition). The Agency worked with general practitioner surgeries, pharmacies and several community groups in areas with large populations of older people to ensure that the message reached as many people as possible. Posters and leaflets were produced, and information boxes were printed on several million pharmacy paper bags used for dispensing prescriptions. Public health education campaigns are also taking place in other European countries, Australia, Canada, New Zealand and the USA (for weblinks to their consumer advice on *Listeria*, see end of chapter). The success of these campaigns is yet to be assessed.

Chapter 6 Exercises: The humble sandwich

Exercise 1: Sandwiches and their fillings

Millions of pre-packed and loose sandwiches are sold every year by retailers, restaurants, sandwich bars, cafés and from vending machines. They can be made from many different types of bread and fillings and are sold chilled or hot. List the potential hazards associated with eating the five sandwich examples below and suggest some 'safer' alternative fillings. Then list another five examples of sandwiches that you have eaten or seen for sale and assess their risk factors and possible alternative fillings. The first row in the table shows you the type of answer that is expected. You may refer to the Microbial CVs in this chapter and Chapter 5 to help you decide which fillings are more risky than others.

Sandwich	Potential hazards	Alternative filling
Bagel filled with cold-smoked salmon, cream cheese and watercress	*Listeria* grows at fridge temperatures and has been isolated from cold-smoked salmon and unpasteurized cheese; watercress may be contaminated with enteric (gut) bacteria such as VTEC	Hot-smoked or canned salmon. Wash watercress thoroughly or replace with thinly sliced onion. Always use pasteurized cream cheese
Baguette with tuna, cucumber and mayonnaise with flat-leaf parsley and spring onions		
Club sandwich made with toasted white bread, smoked ham, sliced cheddar, mayonnaise and lettuce		
Egg and cress with mayonnaise on brown bread		
Falafel, hummus and coriander in pita bread		

continued ➢

Sandwich	Potential hazards	Alternative filling
Hot wrap with Mexican chicken and jalapeño peppers		
Add your own sandwich examples here:		

Exercise 2: Should sandwiches sold in a hospital café be made by volunteers?

You are a manager who has to decide between two systems of production of sandwiches for a hospital café. One system is 'cheap and cheerful' and relies on a team of dedicated and hard-working volunteers from a local charity. The second system is more expensive and involves using a medium-sized local supplier of pre-packed sandwiches.
Before you make your decision, read the following two summaries:

- Members of a local charity who had made sandwiches at a regional UK hospital for many years were asked to leave because of a new European food-hygiene rule. The hospital manager said that all sandwiches must be pre-packed, and the 68 volunteers at the hospital were no longer needed. A spokesman for the charity said it wanted to protect its volunteers from possible prosecution under the Food Safety Act (1990). The volunteers protested, arguing that they had never had an incident of food poisoning in their café. (Adapted from *The Telegraph*, 20 May 1999.)
- An outbreak of listeriosis occurred in the Swindon area of the UK in autumn 2003. Five cases were detected in pregnant women over a 2-month period. The cases were not fatal but the patients suffered prolonged 'flu'-like symptoms with fever and their newborn babies tested positive for *Listeria*. Four of the women had eaten pre-packed sandwiches from a retail outlet in a hospital that they had attended for antenatal appointments. Samples of food and environmental swabs taken from the local supplier of the pre-packed sandwiches revealed the presence of *Listeria monocytogenes* in a brie and cranberry sandwich and on the chopping boards, the sink plug holes and a cleaning sponge. The sandwich supplier closed down voluntarily. (Adapted from *Eurosurveillance Monthly*, 11 (6), June 2006.)

continued ➢

Use the following table to list the potential hazards linked with the two methods of sandwich making.

Risk factors associated with sandwich making	
Sandwiches made by volunteers	**Pre-packed sandwiches from commercial supplier**

Taking all of the above risk factors into consideration, which of the two methods of making sandwiches would you select for the hospital café?

Exercise 3: Complying with the law

In January 2006, a European Regulation on Microbiological Criteria for Foods came into force. This law recommends that food businesses manufacturing ready-to-eat foods that could pose a risk to public health through the presence or growth of *L. monocytogenes* should monitor processing areas and equipment for the presence of this organism as part of their sampling plans. In addition, if the food is to be stored for a specified number of days (shelf life) prior to consumption, then *L. monocytogenes* should not exceed 100 bacteria/g during this period. If this cannot be guaranteed, then it should be absent from 25 g of the food when it leaves the food business operator.
Consider these questions:

- Would knowledge of the law change your decision made in Exercise 2?
- Do you think that this law helps to prevent *Listeria* outbreaks?
- Discuss your answers with other students on your course.

References and further reading

Advisory Committee on the Microbiological Safety of Food (ACMSF). *Report on the increased incidence of listeriosis in the UK (2010)* (available from: **http://www. food. gov. uk/multimedia/pdfs/committee/acmsflisteria. pdf**).

Bell, C and Kyriyakides, A (2005). Listeria*: A practical approach to the organism and its control*, 2nd edn. Wiley-Blackwell, London.

Pennington, TH (1998). *The Pennington Group Report on the circumstances leading to the 1996 outbreak of infection with* E. coli *O157 in central Scotland, the implications for food safety and the lessons to be learned.* The Stationery Office, Edinburgh.

Pennington, TH (2000) VTEC: lessons learned from British outbreaks. *Journal of Applied Microbiology* Symposium Supplement, **88**, 90S–98S (available from: **http://www. food. gov. uk/multimedia/pdfs/publication/ecolifactsheet0211. pdf**).

Pennington, TH (2009) *The public inquiry into the September 2005 outbreak of E. coli O157 in South Wales* (available from: **http://www. ecoliinquirywales. org**).

Weatherill, S (on behalf of the Canadian Government)(2009). *Report of the independent investigator into the 2008 listeriosis outbreak* (available from: **http://www. listeriosis-listeriose. investigation-enquete. gc. ca/lirs_rpt_e. pdf**).

Weblinks

Food Standards Agency (2011). *E. coli* O157 control of cross-contamination. Guidance document for food-business operators and enforcement authorities (available from:
http://www. food. gov. uk/multimedia/pdfs/publication/ecoliguide0211. pdf).

and

http://www.food.gov.uk/multimedia/pdfs/enforcement/ crosscontaminationqanda.pdf

E. coli *O157: An invisible threat to your business.* Food Standards Agency factsheet (available from:
http://www. food. gov. uk/multimedia/pdfs/publication/ecolifactsheet0211. pdf)

Chilled Food Association (2010). *Shelf life of ready to eat food in relation to* Listeria monocytogenes – *Guidance for food-business operators* (available from: **http:// www. chilledfood. org**).

For consumer advice on listeriosis:

UK

http://eatwell. gov. uk/healthissues/foodpoisoning/abugslife/

http://nhs. uk/conditions/Listeriosis/

http://www. hpa. org. uk/Publications/InfectiousDiseases/Factsheets/factListeria/

Australia and New Zealand

http://www. foodstandards. gov. au/_srcfiles/Listeria. pdf

USA

http://www. fda. gov/Food/ResourcesForYou/HealthEducators/ucm081785. htm

Canada

http://www. inspection. gc. ca/english/fssa/concen/cause/listeriae. shtml

Germany

http://www. bfr. bund. de/cd/10966

7

Clostridia, viruses and other undesirables

In this chapter we examine several important pathogens that food professionals need to be aware of. Some of them, such as *Clostridium perfringens* and norovirus, cause mild disease in comparison with *Salmonella* or *Campylobacter* (Chapter 5) and so are often not reported to public health authorities. Others, like *Clostridium botulinum*, can be as deadly as the verocytotoxin-producing *Escherichia coli* (VTEC) or *Listeria* (Chapter 6) but tend to occur very rarely. Of course, this does not mean that they can be ignored. These pathogens deserve our attention because the illnesses they cause are preventable.

The spore formers: clostridia and bacilli

Ordinary cooking temperatures used to destroy many food-poisoning bacteria such as *Salmonella* don't work with clostridia or bacilli because they form heat-resistant **spores**. From the point of view of the microbe, these hardy structures are an ingenious way of ensuring survival of the species. When environmental conditions are not favourable for growth, bacterial cells known as **mother cells** form spores inside them, often referred to as **endospores** (see Fig. 2.7). The spores have a tough outer coat that protects them from all manner of chemical and physical attack (see Microbial CV for *Clostridium* p. 93). They are resistant to heat, extremes of acidity and alkalinity, chemicals including disinfectants and preservatives, freezing, dehydration and irradiation.

Once released from the mother cell into the environment, bacterial spores can remain dormant for centuries. A fairly strong stimulus or 'jolt' is needed to wake them up from their slumber. Heat shock is one such stimulus. Boiling dormant spores in a food followed by slow cooling induces them to **germinate** or shed their outer coat and start producing young, vigorous **vegetative cells**, which go on to multiply at a remarkably fast rate. Numbers can double every 10 minutes if conditions are right. The vegetative cells then produce toxins (poisons), either in the food itself or in the small intestine of the person eating it, to cause illness.

A key feature of clostridia is that they cannot grow in the presence of air. Even the smallest amount of oxygen in the air can inhibit their growth. The way in which this property can be exploited in food preservation will be discussed in Chapter 8.

Clostridium botulinum

Botulism was first recognized as an illness in the late eighteenth century due to its distinctive and very serious symptoms, often leading to death. The illness was linked with the consumption of certain types of sausages and so was named after *botulus*, the Latin name for sausage. The organism responsible for the illness, *Clostridium botulinum*, was isolated in 1896 by Emile van Ermengem, a former student of Robert Koch (see Box 3.1).

C. botulinum produces one of the deadliest toxins on the planet. It is known as a **neurotoxin** as it blocks the transmission of signals along nerves (neurons) and leads to paralysis and often death (see Microbial CV for *Clostridium*). Seven chemically distinct neurotoxins are recognized but, for the purposes of this book, we will refer to them collectively as botulinum toxin. As little as 30 nanogrammes (ng) of toxin in 0.1 g of food is enough to cause disease. Less than 2 kg of the toxin would be enough to kill every person on Earth. These properties of botulinum toxin have attracted some attention as potentially lethal weapons of mass destruction. But extremely small quantities of the neurotoxin can be beneficial, for example when injected into muscles in the treatment of neurological conditions such as facial muscle spasms. In recent years, the use of the toxin has also become more widespread in cosmetic treatments that allegedly 'iron out' facial wrinkles.

Many strains of clostridia, including *C. botulinum*, are **proteolytic** (able to rapidly degrade proteins) and betray their presence by a rancid smell. When such smells are detected, the food must not be tasted because even a small mouthful can cause illness. Mortality from botulism was historically very high at around 30 per cent but is now around 10 per cent (still a high figure for a foodborne illness) provided that the patient is treated with antitoxin quickly. The recovery rate for people who survive the illness is very slow, often stretching to several months.

Cases of botulism in the UK are relatively rare. The last large outbreak caused by a commercially produced food was in 1989. The 26 cases of illness and one death were linked to hazelnut purée used to flavour yogurt. The purée had not been processed adequately to kill botulinum spores. The handful of cases reported in the UK in the 2000s have mostly been linked with home-preserved foods imported from other countries, for example bottled mushrooms in oil from Italy and pork sausage from Poland.

In Europe, a total of 2388 cases of botulism were reported in the 10-year period from 1995 to 2004; of these, 850 or 36 per cent were in Poland. Home preserving of vegetables and meat is still popular in eastern and southern Europe, particularly in rural areas, and this is reflected in higher incidence of botulism. Outside Europe, the Inuit Indians of North America are at higher risk of botulism due to the practice of preserving fish and meat from beavers and whales in sealed containers buried underground for prolonged periods. Around 30 cases are reported in the USA every year.

Microbial CV *Clostridium*

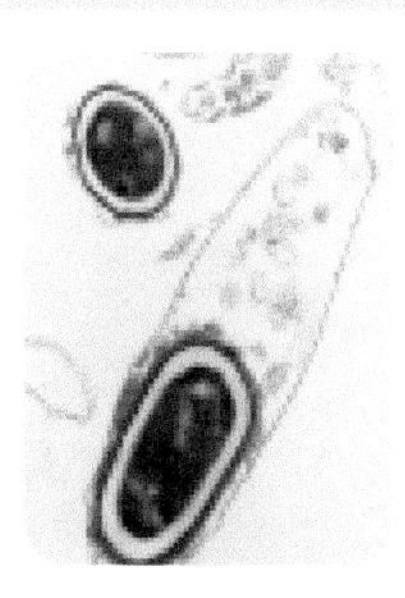

Clostridium botulinum, transmission electron micrograph showing spores inside and out of a cell.

Photo credit: UK Institute of Food Research.

Main address: Soil and sediments at the bottom of rivers, lakes and coastal waters.

Other addresses: Water, intestines of mammals including humans and fish, internal organs of crabs and other shellfish.

Family background: The genus *Clostridium* is large. Many species are harmless but some can kill. In foods, the most deadly species is *Clostridium botulinum* but *Clostridium perfringens* can also cause food poisoning. *C. difficile* is responsible for many hospital-acquired infections while *C. tetani* can infect wounds.

Appearance: All clostridia are Gram-positive rods.

Lifeskills: Most clostridia like it hot, preferably around 45°C but some strains of *C. botulinum* can grow at chill temperatures. All clostridia hate oxygen and form hardy spores that resist drying and boiling. *C. botulinum* produces its toxin in food whilst *C. perfringens* does so after eating, in the small intestine.

Unusual qualities: After surviving boiling, spores can germinate (form new cells) and multiply in slow-cooling food to produce toxins (poisons). Must have oxygen-free conditions to grow.

Mode of transport to human victim:
C. botulinum: poorly processed canned foods that are not acidic (e.g. meat, tuna, soups, vegetables like corn, green beans, mushrooms, olives; home-canned meat and vegetables; vacuum-packed hot-smoked white fish; fermented, lightly smoked fish and seafood; honey; hazelnut purée).

C. perfringens: meat dishes that have been allowed to cool slowly after cooking.

Disease-causing skills: *C. botulinum* produces one of the deadliest neurotoxins (nerve poisons) on Earth. Dry mouth and blurred vision start within a day of eating the affected food. Difficulty in swallowing, speaking and breathing follow and may end in complete paralysis and death from respiratory failure. Recovery is slow and can take 6–8 months.

C. perfringens causes diarrhoea, abdominal pain and nausea within 12–36 hours of eating the contaminated food. Illness rarely lasts longer than a day or two.

Achievements: Botulism can be fatal but is now very rare in many countries. *C. perfringens* is very common but the illness relatively mild, so often goes unreported. The elderly and very young are more vulnerable to both organisms.

Like all clostridia, *C. botulinum* produces very hardy spores but the toxin is sensitive to heat. It can be destroyed by heating to 80°C for at least 10 minutes but this should never be used as a control measure, as the risk of spore survival is too high.

The control of botulism has been achieved largely due to the very strict processing regimes adopted by the canning industry (see Chapter 8). However, as often happens in food technology, new processes have given rise to new risks. For example, vacuum packing of both raw and cooked foods is now commonplace in the food-service industry, as well as in retailing. Consequently, in recent years there has been increased recognition of a group of *C. botulinum* known as **non-proteolytic** strains. Unlike proteolytic strains, whose degrading abilities make foods smell bad, the non-proteolytic strains remain hidden to the detecting powers of the human nose (Box 7.1). Crucially, non-proteolytic *C. botulinum* can grow at chill temperatures down to 3°C while the proteolytic strains require a

Box 7.1 The 'yuk' factor: the protective role of disgust

When faced with a soiled nappy, toenail clippings or rotting meat, most people screw up their faces and cry 'yuk' or 'eugh'! Disgust is a universal human emotion and provokes a familiar facial expression that is recognized across different cultures. Disgust can stop us in our tracks, make us shudder and even induce feelings of nausea. Bodily fluids such as urine, vomit and sweat are considered disgusting by most people. The sight of faeces, blood, discarded condoms, worms and rats can make some people gag. The physiological reaction is instinctive. All of these items have the potential to carry pathogens and so it's been suggested that disgust evolved to protect us from infectious disease.

The apparent protective role of disgust works only up to a point. Food that looks rotten or smells bad is thrown away instinctively. Meat dishes containing high numbers of certain clostridia smell so bad that they are discarded immediately. The problem is that many foodborne pathogens are invisible to the naked eye and produce no smell at all, even when present in very high numbers. In a UK survey of 2300 adults, nearly 60 per cent of respondents claimed that they could tell if food was 'off' by appearance or smell. In another survey, nearly half of the 450 food handlers interviewed made the same claim. This is wrong. Our senses of sight and smell are not sensitive enough to detect microbial pathogens in food and invoke the protective effect of disgust.

Even when we do feel disgust, we sometimes suppress it for social reasons. In polite company, we might force down unpleasant-looking or smelly foods if refusal could cause offence. And what of the chef who caused a major norovirus outbreak in a London restaurant by rinsing the salad leaves he had just vomited over with cold water and then serving them to customers? Was his 'yuk' instinct completely switched off?

Disgust is of little help in protecting us from unsafe food.

minimum of 12°C to grow. Consequently, non-proteolytic *C. botulinum* is a potential hazard in chilled foods sealed in vacuum or modified atmosphere packs. Sporadic cases acquired by eating contaminated vacuum-packed smoked fish have been reported in Sweden, Finland and France. Further details on achieving control under these conditions are given in Chapter 8.

As with many other illnesses caused by foodborne pathogens, the consequences of botulism are more serious in vulnerable groups such as the very young and the elderly. In most adults, the gut microflora competes successfully with *C. botulinum* and prevents it from growing and producing toxin once in the intestine. However, in infants below the age of 12 months, *C. botulinum* can out-compete the immature flora and grow. Several cases of infant botulism have been reported as a result of feeding infants with honey contaminated with botulinum spores. For this reason, giving honey in any form to infants is not recommended.

Clostridium perfringens

As a spore former, *C. perfringens* shares many of the physiological attributes of other clostridia. However, the illness caused by *C. perfringens* is relatively mild

Box 7.2 Two weddings and a caterer

In July 2009, the North West London Health Protection Unit was notified of several cases of gastroenteritis reported by guests attending two separate wedding receptions. The weddings took place on the same day and were supplied by the same caterer.

Investigations revealed that 93 guests experienced diarrhoea, abdominal pain and nausea followed by vomiting, headaches and fever in some of the cases. Symptoms started on average 10 hours after eating at the wedding receptions and the illness lasted 2–3 days. Enterotoxin from *C. perfringens* was detected in stool samples from several patients involved in the outbreak. The illnesses were linked to two curry-based dishes from the buffet-style menu: lamb karahi and jeera chicken.

Environmental health officers visited the caterer's kitchen and discovered high levels of enteric bacteria, indicating poor hygiene, on surfaces and in ingredients, including a garlic and ginger paste, and paneer cheese. A blast chiller was available on the premises but not used appropriately at the time of the outbreak. As a result, many of the meat-based dishes were cooled too slowly after cooking. The vans used to transport food from the kitchens to the wedding venues were not refrigerated and the events took place in July. None of the staff was adequately trained in food hygiene. In addition, hand swabs taken from the chef who had prepared both the lamb karahi and the jeera chicken tested positive for faecal bacteria, indicating poor personal hygiene. Fortunately, in this case, there were no funerals. The caterer was fined and the failures in food-handling practices were rectified.

and short lived and so often goes unreported (see Microbial CV for *Clostridium*). Elderly people are usually more seriously affected. It tends to get more noticed during outbreaks (see Box 7.2). In the UK, the number of outbreaks caused by *C. perfringens* has been around 2–4 per year between 2005 and 2010, affecting some 150 people annually. In such outbreaks, the most common cause is a meat dish that has been prepared too far in advance and kept warm for several hours before serving. As with all relatively mild illnesses, the real figures are likely to be much higher. For example, in the USA, it has been estimated that *C. perfringens* makes up to 1 million people ill every year.

Bacilli

Like the clostridia, bacilli are spore formers that may contaminate foods when they come into contact with soil. *Bacillus cereus*, *B. subtilis* and *B. licheniformis* are all capable of causing human disease but *B. cereus* is the most important.

There are two main types of illness caused by *B. cereus* (Table 7.1).

Table 7.1 Types of illness caused by *Bacillus cereus*

	Diarrhoeal type	Vomiting (or emetic) type
Incubation	8–16 hours	1–5 hours
Symptoms	Diarrhoea, abdominal pain, sometimes nausea	Nausea, vomiting, sometimes diarrhoea
Duration of illness	12–24 hours	6–24 hours
Toxin properties	Can be destroyed by heating at 56°C for 5 minutes	Cannot be destroyed even after heating at 126°C for 90 minutes!
Foods affected	Meat products, soups and sauces	Starchy foods such as rice (boiled, fried and in puddings), pasta, baked potato

As the illness is relatively mild, patients rarely visit their doctor and cases are often not reported to national surveillance schemes. In the UK, the number of reported cases of food poisoning by *Bacillus* spp. has been below 50 per year since the turn of the millennium but the actual number in the community is likely to be much higher.

B. stearothermophilus is, as the name suggests, a very heat-resistant species. Fortunately, it does not cause food poisoning but can be a nuisance as a spoilage agent of canned foods. The microbe produces large amounts of gas during growth and has been known to make tins of food explode.

Control measures for bacilli are the same as for the clostridia and are described in Chapter 8.

Staphylococcus aureus

Human skin is inhabited by two species from the genus *Staphylococcus*: *S. epidermidis* and *S. aureus*. Both microbes are part of the normal skin flora. *S. epidermidis* is harmless but *S. aureus* can cause disease if the skin is broken, as in cuts, wounds and boils, or if it is transferred to foods where it can grow and produce toxin. It is for this reason that outbreaks of staphylococcal food poisoning are often linked with poor personal hygiene.

Estimates vary but about 30 per cent of the human population are carriers of *S. aureus*. Like Typhoid Mary (Box 5.1), carriers show no symptoms of illness but can spread the organism to food or other people. As shown in Fig. 7.1, the human nose is a favourite haunt of *S. aureus* in carriers and the general population alike. Humans habitually scratch, pick and blow their noses so it is not surprising that *S. aureus* is frequently isolated from fingers and hands. People not only carry staphylococci but they also shed them into the environment around them. Some carriers are so heavily colonized that they are followed by a cloud of tiny skin particles, each one with a few staphylococcal passengers attached to it.

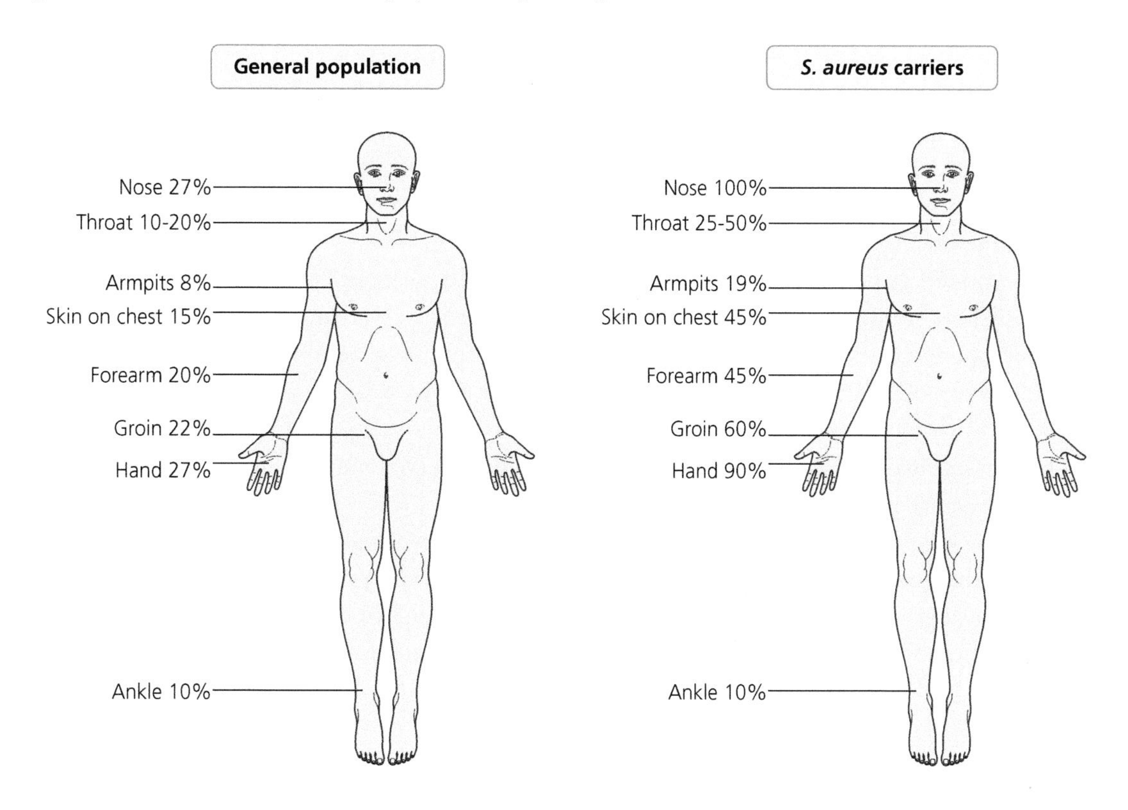

Figure 7.1 People carry staphylococci. *Staphylococcus aureus* can be isolated much more frequently from body parts of healthy carriers than from the general population. Percentages indicate the frequency of isolation from each body part. Adapted from Wertheim *et al.* (2005).

Box 7.3 Features of *Staphylococcus aureus* infection

Incubation	1–6 hours
Symptoms	Nausea, vomiting, diarrhoea, abdominal pain
Duration of illness	24 hours
Toxin properties	Relatively heat resistant, degrades slowly on prolonged boiling

Some carriers harbour methicillin-resistant *Staphylococcus aureus* (MRSA). Hospital-acquired MRSA is very serious if it enters the body and can be life threatening.

As shown in Box 7.3, foodborne *S. aureus* infection is relatively mild and often goes unreported. In severe cases, particularly in the elderly, infants and the infirm, treatment for dehydration may be necessary.

As shown in Figs 2.4 and 2.6, *S. aureus* is Gram positive and spherical in shape. Like *Salmonella* and *Campylobacter*, *S. aureus* is readily destroyed by heat but the toxin persists even after prolonged cooking.

S. aureus grows best at 37°C. It requires a minimum temperature of 7°C to grow and 10°C to produce toxin. Staphylococci are very hardy and resistant to fluctuations in temperature and humidity. The bacteria survive readily on dust particles, paper, mops, formica table tops, fabrics and plastics. All objects touched by human hands harbour *S. aureus*, from pens, phones and computer keyboards to uniforms, curtains and men's ties (see Chapter 3 for more examples of surfaces often contaminated with bacteria).

S. aureus prefers protein-rich, low-acid foods such as cooked meats and poultry, cooked fish and seafoods and dairy products. Products such as cream-filled pastries, chocolate éclairs, trifle and cream cakes are often implicated in outbreaks, especially when stored at room temperature in the summer months. *S. aureus* can grow in very salty foods, even those containing as much as 20 per cent salt. Hence it has been associated with ham, corned beef, tongue and preserved meats where other bacteria don't grow.

More than half of all outbreaks have been linked with catering premises, especially in the summer months when temperature control of foods prepared for large functions may be difficult. Poor personal hygiene, contaminated equipment and temperature abuse are often linked together in outbreaks of *S. aureus* poisoning.

Yersinia enterocolitica

This bacterium causes typical gastrointestinal illness as shown in Box 7.4. Vulnerable groups suffer more severe symptoms that can lead to complications such as arthritis. The highest burden of disease is in children below the age of 15 years. Severe

Box 7.4 Features of *Yersinia enterocolitica* infection

Incubation	1–10 days
Symptoms	Diarrhoea, fever and abdominal pain
Duration of illness	Symptoms subside after 2–4 days but may persist, in a milder form, for up to 2 weeks
Toxin properties	Relatively heat resistant, degrades slowly on prolonged boiling

abdominal pain caused by *Yersinia* in children is sometimes mistaken for appendicitis. The organism is foodborne but can also spread from person to person.

In the first decade of the millennium, fewer than 100 laboratory-confirmed cases of illness caused by *Y. enterocolitica* were reported in the UK per year. However, this is probably a gross underestimate due to the fact that clinical laboratories don't routinely test for *Yersinia*. In the USA, this microbe is thought to be responsible for up to 100 000 cases of illness per year. In Europe, nearly 8200 confirmed cases of yersiniosis were reported in 2008.

This Gram-negative organism has been isolated from many environmental sources, including water from lakes and rivers, as well as wild and domestic animals, especially pigs.

Y. enterocolitica is one to watch because, like *Listeria*, it can grow at refrigeration temperatures. For example, 21 people were sickened in Norway after eating radicchio rosso from a refrigerated, bagged salad mix. Although it grows fastest at 22–29°C, its full temperature range is from 0 to 45°C. Foods frequently responsible for yersiniosis are milk and dairy products, raw pork and pork products.

Vibrio spp.

The most infamous species in the *Vibrio* genus is *Vibrio cholerae*, responsible for causing cholera. This short, sharp illness can be fatal within hours and has caused many devastating epidemics since antiquity. Public health measures such as water and sewage sanitation have ensured that cholera is now relatively rare in the developed world. In developing countries, cholera is still common and epidemics strike regularly when natural disasters such as earthquakes destroy water and sewage treatment facilities.

The main foodborne member of the *Vibrio* genus is *Vibrio parahaemolyticus*. The disease caused by this organism has sometimes been described as a mild form of cholera (Box 7.5).

Like all vibrios, *V. parahaemolyticus* is Gram negative and distinctively comma shaped (see Fig. 2.4). It is a salt-loving organism found naturally in coastal and estuarine seawater.

Box 7.5 Features of *Vibrio parahaemolyticus* infection

Incubation	2–48 hours (usually 12–18 hours)
Symptoms	Severe diarrhoea often leading to dehydration, abdominal pain, vomiting and fever
Duration of illness	2–5 days

V. parahaemolyticus has been isolated from raw fish, prawns and crabs (Fig 7.3). Outbreaks are relatively rare but one such incident affecting nearly 300 people in Japan was linked with salted sardines. Generally, numbers of bacteria are too low in raw shellfish to cause illness but the organism can grow rapidly in temperature-abused seafoods. The organism is sensitive to cold and so tends to be seasonal, striking mainly in the summer months. It is readily destroyed by heat.

The parasitic protozoa

Several species in the three genera of protozoan parasites *Cryptosporidium*, *Cyclospora* and *Giardia* cause gastroenteritis. The symptoms include classic diarrhoea, abdominal pain, nausea and vomiting. The incubation period is often around 3 days but can be as long as 6 weeks. Symptoms can be more severe in vulnerable groups, lasting up to 6 weeks. For example, infection with *Cryptosporidium* can be life threatening in AIDS patients receiving treatment with immuno-suppressing drugs.

Like the viruses (discussed in more detail in the next section), the protozoa are parasites. They need a host to invade in order to grow and multiply. They do not grow in foods or in the environment. Their life cycles are arguably more complex than those of bacteria. They grow inside their human and animal hosts to reach very high numbers in faeces. Hence, infection occurs when direct contact is made with faeces, or foods and water that have been contaminated with faeces from an infected person. Infected food handlers are often responsible for spreading protozoa.

In 1996, an outbreak of illness caused by *Cyclospora cayetanensis* sickened nearly 1500 people across the USA. The outbreak was traced back to sewage-contaminated raspberries imported from Guatemala. Further outbreaks of similar magnitude and linked to Guatemalan raspberries occurred in the following 2 years across the USA and Canada. It wasn't until strict hygiene standards and seasonal restrictions were imposed by these two countries on Guatemalan berry imports that the outbreaks came under control. Fresh salads and basil have also been implicated in outbreaks in North America and Europe.

In Europe, nearly 170 000 cases of giardiasis were reported in 2008 but 90 per cent of these occurred in Romania. Over 7000 cases of cryptosporidiosis were also reported in the same year but nearly half of the 22 European countries providing data had no cases at all. It is likely that there is substantial under-reporting of cases of these illnesses.

Another protozoan parasite, *Toxoplasma gondii*, can cause a 'flu'-like illness with fever, fatigue and muscle pain but many healthy people show no symptoms of illness. It has been estimated that up to 1 billion people may be infected with the parasite worldwide. In the UK, about 400 cases of toxoplasmosis are diagnosed annually. In the USA, it is estimated that up to 90 000 illnesses may occur every year.

In pregnant women and people with weakened immune systems such as HIV/AIDS patients or organ transplant recipients, toxoplasmosis can be severe and lead to complications. Infected unborn babies may die *in utero* or be born with serious eye and brain defects.

Many mammals and birds are infected with *T. gondii*. The chief culprit is the domestic cat, which can shed millions of microscopic cysts (hardy structures equivalent to spores in bacteria) in its faeces. The cysts can also embed themselves in muscle tissue and remain in the body for many years. Eating undercooked, infected meat (mainly pork and lamb) and cross-contamination with cat faeces are the main modes of transmission to humans.

Viruses

Like many bacteria, the vast majority of viruses that exist on the planet are harmless to humans. A glassful of seawater contains more viruses than there are people on Earth (currently about 7 billion) but most of them are adapted to infect marine creatures, not humans. Similarly, many viruses specialize in attacking plants or animals. Nevertheless, some viruses can cause serious illness in humans and it is these that we need to concern ourselves with in this book.

Viruses are parasitic creatures that need to invade animal, plant or bacterial cells in order to reproduce. Some biologists would argue that viruses are not, strictly speaking, living organisms at all. Without their unwilling hosts, nothing happens. Free-floating viruses are, for all intents and purposes, dead. Some can even form crystals to protect themselves from harsh environments while waiting for a suitable host to come along. But as soon as a host passes by, the sticky outer coating of the virus helps it to attach itself to the surface of the host's cells. In an attempt to defend itself, the cell membrane folds itself around the virus. Once inside, the virus hijacks the cell's machinery to produce millions of copies of itself. This process upsets the host and often kills it. Exhausted by the attack, the cell pops and releases millions of new viruses into the surroundings to await new victims. If the cells are our own, the damage done is what makes us feel ill. Alive, dead or undead, viruses have a profound effect on life on Earth.

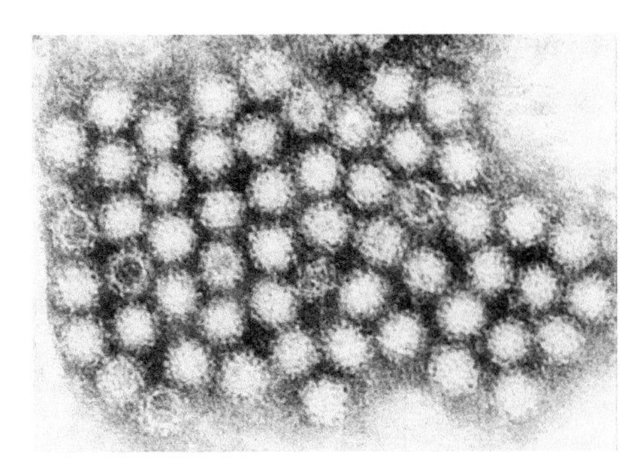

Figure 7.2 Transmission electron micrograph of norovirus showing a spiky outer coat that helps it to stick to and infect human cells. Photo credit: Centers for Disease Control and Prevention (CDC).

Viruses can be thought of as microscopic sacks made of protein and containing one or two strands of deoxyribonucleic acid (**DNA**) or ribonucleic acid (**RNA**). The DNA and RNA are the genetic materials that provide the code for making more viruses. Unlike bacteria, viruses cannot be seen under a light microscope because they are too small. An electron microscope is required to visualize viral structures (see Chapter 2 and Fig. 7.2). As viruses have no cell, they are sometimes referred to as **virus** particles or **virions**.

The two most common foodborne viral pathogens are norovirus and hepatitis A. Both originate from the human gut. Norovirus illness is very common in the developed world but is relatively mild; hepatitis is more common in developing countries and the illness can be severe. Unlike many bacteria such as *Salmonella*, *Campylobacter* and VTEC, norovirus specializes in infecting humans and has no animal reservoir.

Norovirus

Norovirus is a group of viruses formerly known as Norwalk-like viruses, calciviruses or small round structured viruses (SRSVs). Symptoms of viral gastroenteritis usually start 24–48 hours after eating the contaminated food. The symptoms can be alarming. Projectile vomiting can occur suddenly and without warning. Diarrhoea can be explosive and uncontrollable. Varying degrees of nausea, abdominal pain and fever can also occur. The illness lasts for 2–3 days. After the initial uncontrollable onset, the symptoms subside. Some patients may feel weak for up to 3 weeks but generally there are no long-term effects.

Like *Salmonella* (Chapter 5) and *S. aureus* carriers (Fig. 7.1), some people can be carriers of viruses without showing any symptoms of disease. Up to 12 per cent of people in the UK are thought to be shedding low levels of norovirus in their faeces at any one time.

Norovirus is highly infectious and can spread rapidly from person to person as well as via food and the hand-to-mouth route. The infectious dose is very low at around 6–10 virus particles. The virus multiplies rapidly in the intestine so numbers in faeces and vomit can be very high (as many as 10 million per gram). Uncontrollable vomiting can lead to the formation of aerosols (air-borne droplets) that are then inhaled by others in the vicinity or sprayed on to nearby surfaces. Infected food handlers who continue to work while ill have often been implicated in norovirus outbreaks. Semi-closed environments such as hospitals, nursing homes, schools and cruise ships provide ideal conditions for the virus to spread rapidly. In the winter months when windows are closed, the number of cases increases, giving rise to the historic name 'winter vomiting disease'.

The exact numbers of norovirus illness are not known as most people infected with the virus are never formally tested. Some estimates suggest that 600 000 cases of norovirus illness occur each year in the UK but others put the figures nearer 1 million. In the USA, estimates vary between 5.5 and 23 million cases of norovirus illness occurring annually.

The most notorious source of foodborne norovirus outbreaks is the raw oyster (Fig. 7.3). Other shellfish such as mussels, clams and cockles are also often implicated. These shellfish feed by filtering seawater through their gills. If the surrounding water is contaminated with sewage, virus particles can accumulate in their flesh. As oysters and mussels are often eaten raw or very lightly cooked, shellfish farms must be protected from sewage contamination. A purification process known as depuration is sometimes used and involves moving live shellfish from their growing beds to tanks containing clean water for 42 hours before sale. This works well in clearing out faecal bacteria but not norovirus. Norovirus outbreaks caused by 'depurated' shellfish have been reported. Norovirus-contaminated oysters sicken hundreds of people on a regular basis during the winter months.

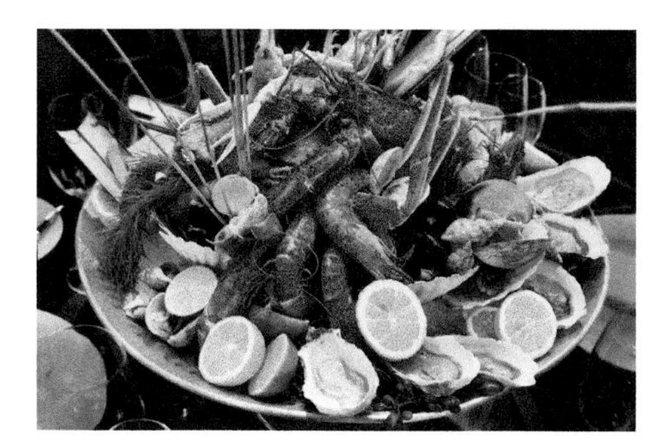

Figure 7.3 Raw oysters, shown in the foreground, are a common source of norovirus. Other shellfish such as prawns, lobster and crab can be contaminated by the bacterium *Vibrio parahaemolyticus* (© Tatiana Kitaeva, Fotolia).

Crops that come into contact with sewage and are eaten raw can also be contaminated with foodborne viruses. For example, in 2005, nearly 600 people in a hospital and a home nursing scheme were made ill in Denmark after eating frozen raspberries imported from Poland and contaminated with norovirus. A cluster of norovirus outbreaks affecting around 200 people in Finland was traced again in 2009 to frozen raspberries from Poland. Lettuce, leafy greens, ice and water have also been linked with norovirus illness. Viral particles persist and retain their ability to infect people on lettuce leaves and slices of ready-to-eat turkey stored at chill temperatures (7°C) for as long as 10 days.

Norovirus can survive heating at 60°C for 10 minutes but are inactivated at temperatures over 65°C or by boiling. Cooking at 70°C for 2 minutes or 85–90°C for 90 seconds also works. The viruses are relatively acid tolerant and so can survive the acidity of soft fruit such as raspberries and strawberries, vinegar and yogurt. They are also not averse to alcohol and high sugar concentrations.

Norovirus survives well on surfaces. A door knob heavily contaminated with viruses from an infected person can be a continuing source of infection even after six people have touched it. Contact with kitchen utensils, work surfaces and even soft furnishings previously handled by an infected person can spread the disease.

Detergent-based cleaning of surfaces using kitchen cloths has no effect on virus survival. A bleach solution can be effective in reducing numbers but does not eliminate the particles completely. The virus is sensitive to ultraviolet (UV) light and it has been suggested that exposure to more hours of sunlight in the summer months may partly explain why the virus is more common in winter. Sewage treatment using UV light may in the future help to reduce levels of viral pollution in river water.

People infected with norovirus can readily transfer the virus on to the foods that they prepare. Foods such as salads, canapés and cakes are particularly vulnerable. The more a food is handled, the more likely it is to become contaminated by infected food handlers. Therefore, the only effective control measure for norovirus is exclusion from work for at least 48 hours after vomiting and diarrhoea have ceased.

In the UK, all packages of oysters are labelled with a 'Healthmark' showing the supplier and batch number, which identifies the oyster bed from which the oysters were harvested. Retailers and caterers are required by law to keep this label for 60 days in case there is an outbreak and the information is needed to trace the source. Factsheets are also available for both the public and food professionals (see weblinks).

Norovirus outbreak at The Fat Duck restaurant, UK

A spate of norovirus outbreaks, all traced to contaminated oysters supplied by a single Colchester fishery, affected several high-quality catering establishments in the UK in 2009. The first outbreak made 14 people ill after eating oysters on the 'aphrodisiac menu' at St Pancras Grand Hotel in London. Another two outbreaks made 14 passengers and four staff members ill after eating raw oysters on the luxury Orient Express train. But the largest norovirus outbreak associated with a restaurant occurred at The Fat Duck, a three Michelin starred establishment run by internationally acclaimed chef Heston Blumenthal. More than 500 people, representing about 15 per cent of the diners at the restaurant, were reported ill during this outbreak. We examine the incident in more detail because of the many lessons that can be learned from it.

The Fat Duck restaurant is famous in the world of fine dining for its unusual dishes prepared using the principles of molecular gastronomy. Concoctions such as 'snail porridge, Joselito ham', 'salmon poached in liquorice gel, artichokes, vanilla mayonnaise and Manni olive oil' and 'nitro-scrambled egg and bacon ice cream, pain perdu, tea jelly' feature on the popular 'tasting menu'. Although an á la carte menu is also on offer, about 90 per cent of the guests choose the tasting menu made up of no less than 16 dishes. Prepared by a small army of chefs, these elaborate dishes are works of art when arranged on a plate. Despite the eye-watering prices, the restaurant is fully booked for months ahead and serves about 1750 customers per month.

In January 2009, the restaurant started receiving complaints from diners who had developed diarrhoea, vomiting and nausea within 24–48 hours of eating a meal. In most cases, the reported symptoms lasted 3 days. These symptoms were consistent with norovirus infection. After receiving 40 such complaints, the restaurant started its own investigation. A private food-safety consultant was hired to audit the restaurant and take samples of dishes for testing by a microbiology laboratory (see timeline in Fig. 7.4). The tests showed no bacteriological problems but the food samples were not tested for viruses.

The restaurant was closed voluntarily and a deep clean of the premises was arranged. A sanitizing agent was used on all surfaces and the carpets were steam-cleaned. Public health authorities were notified of the outbreak shortly after the deep clean. By that stage, the restaurant had received 66 complaints of illness from diners.

A public investigation of the outbreak was initiated and environmental health officers visited the restaurant five times to collect food samples, stool specimens from staff and environmental swabs from a range of surfaces, including the kitchens and toilets. Not surprisingly, all of the 80 environmental swabs taken after the deep clean tested negative for norovirus. By the time the environmental health officers arrived at the restaurant, no fresh foods were left over for testing, so the presence of norovirus in them could not be confirmed. However, statistical analysis of the symptoms, time of onset of the illnesses and foods eaten by sickened diners pointed to contaminated shellfish. Oysters and clams were key ingredients in 'oyster, passion fruit jelly and lavender' and in 'sound of the sea', a dish served

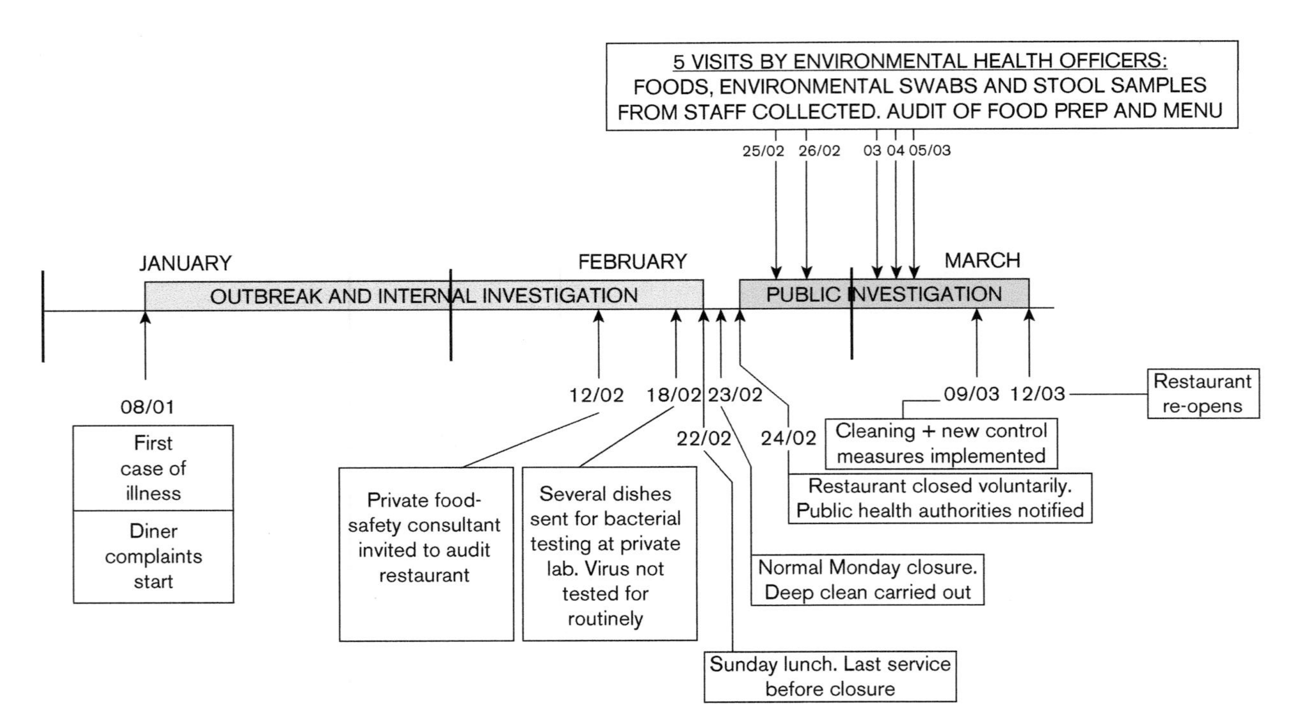

Figure 7.4 Timeline of events during the norovirus outbreak at The Fat Duck restaurant in 2009. Data from Health Protection Agency (HPA), UK.

with an iPod so that the diner can listen to the sound of waves crashing against the seashore while eating. Another dish, the 'jelly of quail, langoustine cream and parfait of foie gras' was affected, albeit to a lesser extent. Further investigation revealed that the oysters had been sourced from Colchester and the razor clams from a fishery in Devon. Samples of shellfish from both suppliers tested positive for norovirus.

Laboratory analyses of stool samples from 10 diners and six staff confirmed the presence of norovirus. At the time of the outbreak, the restaurant employed 57 regular staff and provided work experience for six visiting chefs. All regular staff were interviewed during the public health investigation. It was discovered that 17 staff had symptoms of gastrointestinal illness in January and February. Among these, six continued to work while feeling unwell and nine returned to work less than 48 hours after experiencing gastrointestinal symptoms. One member of staff vomited in the restaurant toilets on a Monday when the business was normally closed. The restaurant's records showed just three members of staff on sickness leave due to gastrointestinal illness during the outbreak.

Although hand-washing facilities were adequate at the restaurant, an alcohol gel was also used in the food preparation areas. The product used was not effective against viruses. The routine cleaning products used were also ineffective against viruses.

The investigation concluded that the norovirus outbreak was probably introduced to the restaurant via contaminated shellfish but persisted for 6 weeks because of ongoing transmission by staff at the restaurant. Several weaknesses were identified in the restaurant's procedures: a delayed response to the incident, staff working when they should have been off sick, and the wrong cleaning products being used (HPA, 2009).

Prior to re-opening, the restaurant took the following actions:

- All stocks and sauces made in the first 3 months of 2009 were thrown away.
- The recipe for the 'sound of the sea' dish was changed to exclude shellfish. The shells used in the presentation of the dish were sanitized between uses as were the iPods providing the sound effects accompanying this dish.
- The number of dishes on the á la carte menu was reduced.
- Cleaning products were changed to include a disinfectant active against viruses.
- A new exclusion period of 72 hours was introduced for staff with symptoms of gastrointestinal illness (the UK Health Protection Agency recommends at least 48 hours exclusion after the last bout of diarrhoea and/or vomiting).
- The training and education of chefs and other staff was intensified with attendance at certified training courses in Hazard Analysis Critical Control Point (HACCP), emphasis on hand-washing regimens and use of educational tools for staff whose first language is not English.

And what of the oyster supplier? The shellfish beds were closed for nearly 3 months to investigate the problem. The investigation concluded that the unusually severe weather patterns and flooding occurring in the period before the outbreak had caused contamination of the shellfish beds with sewage, the prime source of norovirus.

Hepatitis A

Foodborne disease caused by hepatitis A is rare in the developed world. However, hepatitis is much more severe than norovirus infection. Viral hepatitis develops slowly with symptoms appearing 3–6 weeks from eating the contaminated food. In addition to fever and vomiting, the classic symptom of hepatitis is jaundice (yellowing of the eyes and skin) as the liver struggles to cope with the infection. The illness usually lasts several weeks but can be as long as several months.

Hepatitis is much more common in developing countries and is usually linked with drinking untreated water or eating uncooked fruit and vegetables irrigated by sewage-contaminated water. Like norovirus, hepatitis A survives readily in foods and on surfaces but is easily killed by heat. Thorough cooking and disinfection provide efficient means of control, as for norovirus above.

Influenza or 'flu'

Influenza or 'flu' is an infectious disease of humans and animals caused by three types of influenza virus: A, B and C. The flu virus is very contagious and spreads easily from person to person or from animal to animal. Influenza is not a foodborne disease in humans but is mentioned here because several recent epidemics have had devastating effects on food animals including poultry and pigs.

Avian influenza or 'bird flu' viruses have a natural reservoir in wild bird populations. Like all influenza viruses, the avian strains have the ability to change rapidly as they move from one host cell to another. Two different viral strains can infect the same cell and re-arrange their genes to form an entirely new strain. Such new strains have been responsible for causing 24 global bird epidemics since 1959. These bird viruses rarely infect humans and when they do, they cause relatively minor illness.

However, since 1997, a new, more pathogenic strain of avian flu, known as H5N1, has emerged. It started in China and spread westwards from 2003 onwards and eventually reached the Netherlands and the UK. The virus caused huge outbreaks in farm birds and several poultry farms were decimated by the disease in 2007. Fewer than 500 people were also infected, mainly among South-East Asian people who lived in close proximity to domestic poultry. No human cases of H5N1 were reported in Europe. Nevertheless, there was widespread concern about this strain, partly because of its high mortality rate (around 60 per cent) and partly because the worst human pandemic of the twentieth century was caused by another mutated strain of avian influenza. The 1918 flu pandemic is thought to have killed over 50 million people or about six times as many as died in World War I.

So, what does the food handler need to know about bird flu? Bird flu is rare in humans and usually caught by farmers breathing in the virus while handling sick, live birds. The virus is hardy and survives well in raw poultry meat, as well as in faeces, for at least 35 days at 4°C. Freezing preserves the virus for decades. Notably, the avian virus from the 1918 epidemic was isolated in the 1990s from the body of an Inuit woman who had been buried in the Alaskan permafrost for 75 years! Like other viruses, the bird flu virus survives on surfaces for several weeks. Heating to 70°C kills the virus in seconds. Consequently, thorough cooking and good kitchen and personal hygiene can minimize what is already a low risk of catching avian flu.

Box 7.6 Microbiology Hall of Fame: **WHO and the eradication of smallpox**

On 8 May 1980, the 33rd World Health Assembly of the World Health Organization (WHO) declared that smallpox, a deadly viral disease recognized since the days of the Egyptian Pharaohs, had been eradicated globally. For the first time in human history, a serious illness had been conquered. All that remained to be done was to decide whether or not to destroy the last stocks of the organism held by a handful of national reference laboratories. In the months that followed, new public health campaigns to eliminate polio, malaria, leprosy and rabies were proposed. But to this day, smallpox remains the only disease that has been successfully eradicated worldwide. So, why can't the same approach be used to eradicate other disease-causing organisms, including foodborne pathogens?

The smallpox virus had a number of weaknesses that made it particularly suitable for eradication. A vaccine had been developed that gave long-lasting protection after just a single dose. Furthermore, the vaccine was cheap to produce and heat stable, even in tropical conditions. Crucially, the smallpox virus was so highly adapted to the human body that it could not infect any other animal, whether domestic or wild. The lack of an animal reservoir meant that the spread of the organism was easier to control. Finally, the stable and highly specialist nature of the smallpox virus contributed to its downfall. Most other viral pathogens change rapidly to adapt to new environments. A case in point is HIV, which has already developed resistance to several drugs used to treat AIDS patients. With all its weaknesses, the smallpox virus almost escaped eradication and it was thanks to the extraordinary perseverance of healthcare staff in the field that it eventually succeeded. The eradication of smallpox was a prime example of a successful team effort.

Unfortunately, few pathogens share the same weaknesses with smallpox. It is therefore unlikely that many infectious diseases will be eradicated in the future in the way that smallpox was.

In 2009, the focus of attention shifted from avian flu to another strain of influenza, H1N1. The strain was initially named swine flu because it was genetically similar to pig viruses but it turned out to contain a mixture of genetic material from avian, pig and human strains. The new strain of H1N1 emerged in Mexico and spread very rapidly around the world causing 11 000 cases in 42 countries in the first 4 weeks. The World Health Organization (WHO) declared a global flu pandemic. The strain spread by the respiratory route and was not foodborne. Fortunately, the disease caused by the virus was relatively mild and after an initial surge, the numbers of cases did not reach the figures that were predicted. Like all viruses, the swine flu virus is constantly changing by mutating regularly inside its host, so emergence of a new strain in the future would not be surprising.

Prions

> 'When you have eliminated the impossible, whatever remains,
> however improbable, must be the truth.'
>
> *Sir Arthur Conan Doyle, creator of the fictional detective Sherlock Holmes, 1859–1930*

Creutzfeld–Jakob Disease (CJD) is a very rare but fatal illness affecting mainly elderly people. It usually starts with psychiatric symptoms, followed by slurred speech, tremors and loss of balance. The patient becomes progressively more demented and eventually dies. There is no cure. A similar disease known in Papua New Guinea as *kuru* or 'trembling' disease was described in the 1950s and linked to a tribal ritual of eating the dead bodies of relatives.

In the 1990s a new form of CJD started to appear in the UK, affecting mainly people in their 20s and 30s. This illness was named variant CJD (vCJD). Nearly 80 per cent of all cases of vCJD have occurred in the UK. As of May 2011, 175 cases, of which all but four have died, have been recorded.

The recognition of vCJD as a foodborne disease came during a major and economically devastating outbreak of bovine spongiform encephalopathy (BSE) or 'mad cow disease' in cattle. BSE is the bovine version of a neurological disease with similar symptoms to human CJD. The affected cows become nervous, agitated and develop involuntary jerking movements, lose weight and eventually die. A similar disease also occurs in sheep and goats and is known as scrapie because of the itching and scratching behaviour displayed by the sick animals. All these illnesses are caused by infectious prions. In the late 1980s the requirements for processing animal feed based on recycled carcasses were relaxed allowing prions to survive and cause a massive nationwide epidemic in cattle. What was not appreciated until 1996 was the apparent ability of bovine prions to cause vCJD in humans who ate beef from infected animals.

The BSE outbreak was eventually brought under control by slaughtering and burning hundreds of thousands of the infected cattle and changing animal feeding and slaughtering practices. Feeding cattle with recycled animal meat and bone meal was banned and new procedures for removing neurological tissues such as spinal cord and brain from carcasses during butchering were introduced. The measures were effective and BSE now occurs rarely in the UK. Following a peak of 28 cases in 2000, the numbers of vCJD cases have also decreased. In the years between 2008 and 2010, one to three cases of vCJD per year have been reported in the UK.

So what exactly are prions? The answer is still being debated! If viruses challenge the conventional definition of life, then prions throw it into complete disarray. Prions are proteins that are infectious but are unlike any of the bacteria or viruses described in this book. Prions have no DNA or RNA or other form of nucleic acid that normally provides a genetic blueprint for reproduction. On contact, prions change the structures of normal proteins, causing them to become abnormal and accumulate in the brain. Sometimes referred to as the 'kiss of death', this conversion gives the brain a 'spongy' appearance (hence the name 'spongiform'). The exact way in which this happens is still not well understood.

Prions are everywhere. They have been isolated from grass and many body fluids. They are resistant to boiling. Very high temperature treatments are required to destroy prions, for example 121°C for 1 hour or 134°C for 18 minutes. They are highly resistant to chlorine-based disinfectants.

In Chapters 4–7, we have learned a great deal about the characteristics of the main pathogens responsible for foodborne diseases. In Chapter 8, we move on to the methods available to control them.

Chapter 7 Exercise

You are the manager of a restaurant serving 70 covers twice a day, 6 days per week. During a lunch service, the chef responsible for preparing salads informs you that he's been sick in the staff washroom. What do you do?

Chapter 7 Quiz

1 Which of the following is most likely to cause food poisoning?
  a Tinned sardines.
  b Cooked cod fillet in parsley sauce, served piping hot.
  c A platter of fresh seafood, including raw oysters.
  d Prawn cocktail made with bottled mayonnaise and garnished with lettuce.
  e Tuna and pasta bake, served piping hot.

2 If food is contaminated with food-poisoning bacteria, you can normally tell by:
  a Tasting it – it will taste 'off'.
  b Looking at it – it will look spoiled.
  c Smelling it – it will smell bad.
  d None of the above.
  e I don't know.

3 *Staphylococcus aureus* bacteria are most likely to cause food poisoning when present in which food/beverage?
  a Contaminated water from a lake.
  b A cream cake left overnight at room temperature.
  c Undercooked lamb roast.
  d Lightly cooked fried eggs.
  e I don't know.

4 Name three groups of food-poisoning bacteria that are easily controlled (killed) by heat.

5 You've been served a thoroughly cooked chicken from a farm recently infected with 'bird flu'. Would you eat it? Explain your answer.

References and further reading

Health Protection Agency (2009). *Foodborne illness at The Fat Duck restaurant.* Report of an investigation of a foodborne outbreak of norovirus among diners at The Fat Duck restaurant, Bray, Berkshire, in January and February 2009. Available from: **http://www. hpa. org. uk/web/HPAwebFile/HPAweb_C/1252514873165**

Walker, E, Pritchard, C and Forsythe, S (2003). Food handlers' knowledge in small food businesses. *Food Control* **14**, 339–43.

Wertheim, HFL, Melles, DC, Vos, MC *et al.* (2005). The role of nasal carriage in *Staphylococcus aureus* infections. *Lancet Infectious Diseases* **5**, 751–62.

Four articles on foodborne botulism in Europe in 2011 can be downloaded from the free online journal Eurosurveillance, Vol. 16, Issue 49, 8.12.11, at: **http://www. eurosurveillance.org/ViewArticle.aspx?ArticleId=20033**

Weblinks

Food Standards Agency advice on oysters:
http://www. food. gov. uk/news/newsarchive/2011/jan/oysters

Much additional information is available by searching the Food Standards Agency website:
http://www. food. gov. uk

Many organizations and businesses have produced guidelines on handling live oysters. One of the many examples is available from:
http://www. foodalert. com/newsletter/guidance%20on%20Handling%20 of%20Live%20Oysters. pdf

The Institute of Food Science and Technology has published a useful information statement on *Avian influenza and food* in 2007 followed by updated web pages at:
http://www. ifst. org/science_technology_resources/for_food_professionals/ information_and_news/avian_flu/

Also see the European Food Safety Authority website at:
http://www. efsa. europa. eu

8

Control

After reading Chapters 4–7 as well as the summary in Table 8.1, you could be forgiven for thinking that eating anything at all is a very risky activity. Virtually any food that has not been previously sterilized can, in principle, be a source of food-poisoning organisms once brought into the kitchen or food-processing hall. With so many microbes all around us, how is it possible to control those that may harm us without having an encyclopaedic knowledge of microbiology?

Fortunately, many microbes including the pathogens described in previous chapters share several important characteristics, making it easier to develop common and effective control measures against them. In this chapter, we examine the main control measures available to us.

It is technically possible to produce a food supply consisting entirely of germ-free, sterilized products. The early astronauts flying into space in the 1960s were confident that their food was safe and nutritionally sound but they had to endure bite-sized cubes, freeze-dried powders and purées in toothpaste-like squeezable tubes for days. Food-product development for space flights has come a long way since then. International Space Shuttle crew members of the twenty first century selected their daily menus from a range of 200 food items, many of which looked much like the reheatable ready-made dishes in plastic pouches available from terrestrial supermarkets. Interspersed with the occasional delivery of fresh fruit from Earth, this kind of feeding keeps the astronauts nourished for several months. But, however safe and nutritious it may be, eating in space is no fine-dining experience. The astronauts return to Earth craving for the aromas, textures and flavours that we take for granted and the huge variety of foods that characterize even the simplest of human diets.

So how do we achieve control over microbes without making our foods unpalatable? Absolute safety of food that is both nutritious and enjoyable is impossible to guarantee. However, it is possible to achieve better control over food preparation and reduce the risks currently associated with everyday eating and drinking.

Safe foods don't have to be sterile. Making safe foods is about identifying high-risk ingredients, sites and situations and targeting control measures such as cooking and cleaning appropriately. In other words, we cook and clean when it is

Table 8.1 Main food groups and some of the pathogens commonly associated with them

Food group	Examples	Main human pathogens
Poultry	Chicken, turkey, duck and other poultry meat Eggs	*Campylobacter* and *Salmonella* *Clostridium perfringens* *Salmonella*
Red meat	Beef, pork and lamb	*Salmonella* VTEC *Clostridium perfringens* *Yersinia enterocolitica* *Toxoplasma gondii* *Trichinella spiralis* (in pork)
Cooked, refrigerated, ready-to-eat deli meats	Sliced ham, tongue, bologna, frankfurters Fermented meats (e.g. salami, chorizo)	*Listeria monocytogenes* *Salmonella* VTEC
Dairy products	Milk, cream, yogurt, cheese	*Campylobacter* and *Salmonella* *Listeria monocytogenes* VTEC *Staphylococcus aureus*
Fish	Fresh and frozen fish Ready-to-eat smoked fish	*Clostridium botulinum* Helminth parasites *Listeria monocytogenes*
Shellfish	Oysters, clams, mussels	Norovirus and hepatitis A *Vibrio* *Shigella* *Cryptosporidium*
Fresh produce that is eaten raw	Fruit, lettuce, herbs, salad vegetables	*Salmonella*, VTEC, *Shigella* *Listeria monocytogenes* *Yersinia enterocolitica* Norovirus and hepatitis A Parasitic protozoa: *Cryptosporidium*, *Cyclospora*, *Giardia* *Toxoplasma gondii*
Starchy foods Cooked meat, poultry, vegetable dishes	Cooked rice Casseroles	*Bacillus cereus* *Clostridium perfringens*
Under-processed canned and bottled foods	Home-made bottled vegetables and meats, vegetables and herbs in oil	*Clostridium botulinum*
Chilled processed foods	Chilled ready meals in vacuum or modified atmosphere packing	*Clostridium botulinum*

VTEC, verocytotoxin-producing *Escherichia coli*.

necessary and where it matters in order to reduce exposure to microbes that could be harmful.

How do microbes grow and multiply?

Before we can control microbes, we need to know something about how they grow.

You don't need two bacteria to start a population explosion. One is enough! To ensure survival of each species, the legendary Noah took two of each animal on his Ark, one male and one female. But this would be unnecessary for bacteria because they multiply by splitting themselves into two, a process known as **binary fission**. When a bacterium grows to its maximum size, it forms an inner membrane down the middle of the cell to allow it to split into two cells. An example of a dividing cell is shown in the Microbial CV for *Campylobacter* (Chapter 5). Most yeast cells multiply by a slightly more complex mechanism involving **budding**. Instead of splitting in two equal halves, yeast cells produce a bud, much like flower buds on the branch of a tree. The bud grows while still attached to the mother cell and breaks off when mature enough to survive on its own. Viral replication is very different from that of bacteria and yeasts and is described in Chapter 7, p. 101.

Under ideal conditions, some bacteria can divide into two every 10 minutes. The time to complete one round of cell division is known as the **doubling time**. The consequences of this are illustrated in Fig. 8.1. Given the ideal conditions for

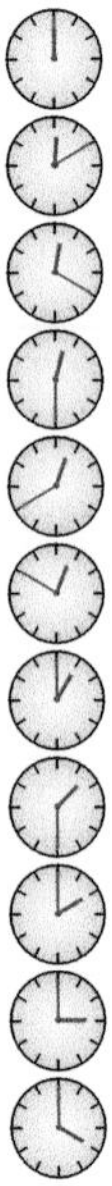

Time	Clock	Number of Microbes	Time elapsed
12:00 (noon)		1	0
12:10 hours		2	10 minutes
12:20		4	20 minutes
12:30		8	30 minutes
12:40		16	40 minutes
12:50		32	50 minutes
13:00		64	1 hour
13:30		512	1½ hours
14:00		4096	2 hours
15:00		262 144	3 hours
16:00		16 777 216 (over 16 million)	4 hours

Figure 8.1 Under ideal conditions, some microbes can multiply and double in number every 10 minutes.

growth, a bacterium with a doubling time of 10 minutes can multiply from one organism to more than 16 million (the equivalent of twice the population of London) in just 4 hours.

Microbial numbers in foods and the environment can be very high, often running to hundreds of thousands or even tens of millions per gram. Writing out all the zeros can be tiresome and impractical, so the numbers are abbreviated mathematically as follows:

100 000 bacteria = 10^5 or 1×10^5

150 000 bacteria = 1.5×10^5

200 000 bacteria = 2×10^5

1 000 000 bacteria (1 million bacteria) = 10^6 or 1×10^6

In this way, some of the large numbers in Fig. 8.1 can be expressed as:

4096 bacteria = 4.096×10^3 This is usually rounded to 4.0×10^3

262 144 bacteria = 2.6×10^5

16 777 216 bacteria = 1.7×10^7

A population of bacteria doesn't always grow and multiply at the same speed. Imagine a bacterium that has just 'landed' in a food from the environment. Before it can start dividing, it needs to adapt to the new surroundings, repair any cellular damage and switch on the metabolic machinery that will drive division and multiplication. Like an athlete before a race, the bacterium 'warms up' during the **lag phase.** This is illustrated in Fig. 8.2.

Following the lag phase, the bacteria multiply rapidly. This is known as the logarithmic or **log phase**, or sometimes as the exponential phase. This rapid growth, represented in Fig. 8.2 as an ever-increasing curve, can't go on forever. The cells eventually use up all the available nutrients or accumulate too many waste

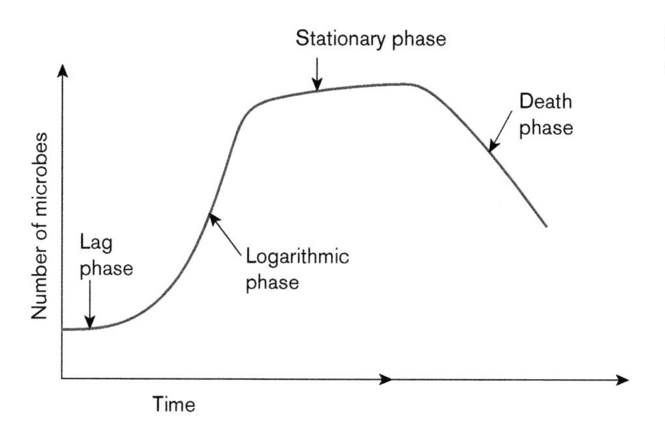

Figure 8.2 A typical microbial growth curve.

products or simply run out of space. During the **stationary phase**, the cells stop dividing but they are still metabolically active. Some species produce toxins or spores during this phase. Eventually, the population starts dying off naturally during the **death phase**. The length of all these phases can vary enormously and depends on the organism itself and the conditions of the environment that it finds itself in.

Under ideal growth conditions, bacteria can reach enormous numbers. In some foods, 10^9 or 1 000 000 000 bacteria per gram are not unusual and some populations can reach even higher levels than that. Furthermore, the shape of the log phase curve makes it difficult to manipulate and interpret the numbers. Therefore, an additional mathematical shortcut is needed. It is necessary to convert these high numbers into logarithms, as follows:

1 000 000 bacteria = 10^6

The logarithm of 1 000 000 is 6

6 500 000 bacteria = 6.5×10^6

The logarithm of 6 500 000 = 6.8

In pre-calculator days, it was necessary to look up logs of numbers in booklets of printed logarithmic tables. This is no longer necessary as most modern calculators, computers and mobile phones have built-in logarithmic functions.

When the logarithms of the numbers used to draw the curve in Fig. 8.2 are plotted on a line graph, a straight line is obtained, as illustrated in Fig. 8.3(a). A similar approach can be used to plot the death of microbes, as shown in Fig. 8.3(b). These principles apply to both pathogenic and spoilage microbes.

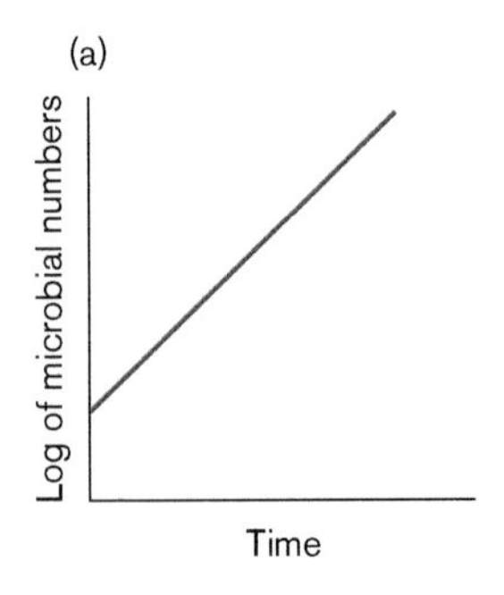

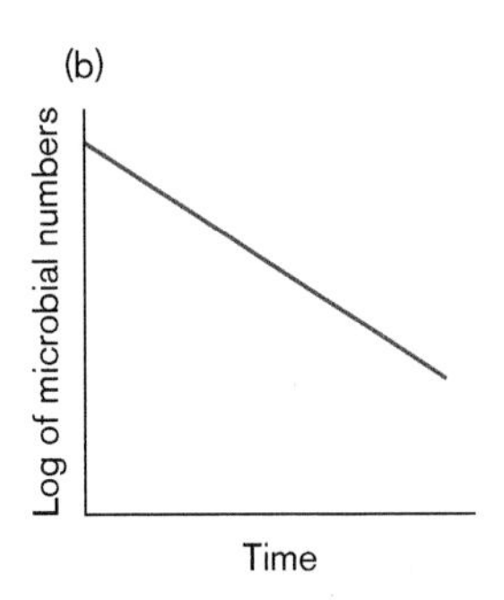

Figure 8.3 Log numbers of microbes plotted against time during rapid growth (a) and death (b).

Control of microbes in foods is dependent on a fine balance between the processing conditions (e.g. cooking), the chemical and physical properties of the food (e.g. acidity and salt content), and its packaging and storage conditions (e.g. refrigeration). We will learn about these in the next sections of this chapter.

Strategies for control

There are two main approaches to achieving microbial control in food. The first is to destroy or *kill all the microbes* present by **sterilization**. This can be done using methods such as incineration or gamma-irradiation. Incineration, of course, destroys the food itself as well as the microbes within it, so there is nothing left to eat. Gamma-irradiation is extremely effective as a means of sterilizing foods such as chicken and spices but is perceived by the consumer as an unacceptable technology and so has not been adopted widely. Sterilization methods are useful occasionally but are neither practical nor desirable for everyday food preparation and processing.

The second approach is to destroy or *kill some of the microbes present and prevent the rest from growing fast* by making the conditions less than ideal for microbial growth. Below we examine killing techniques first and then look at ways of slowing down microbial growth.

Killing techniques

Heating

Heating is the oldest method of killing microorganisms. We cook foods not only to kill microorganisms but also to improve digestibility and palatability. Heating during cooking can take many forms:

- baking
- boiling
- frying
- grilling
- blanching
- toasting.

Sensitivity to heat varies hugely between different microorganisms. In general, bacterial spores are most heat resistant. The spores and cysts of yeasts, moulds and parasites are less heat resistant than bacterial spores. Vegetative cells of bacteria, yeasts and moulds are most heat sensitive. But this rough-and-ready guide is insufficient to help us decide exactly how long and at what temperature foods should be heated.

Because heat is so useful in controlling microbes, a more precise measure of killing efficiency is needed. Such a measure is provided by the decimal reduction time or the D value.

The D value for any given microbe is defined as:

time required at a fixed temperature to kill 90 per cent (or 1 log) of the microorganisms present.

The temperature of the D value is often given as a subscript. For example, a D value obtained at 65°C is written as D_{65}.

D values are measured in carefully controlled experiments and calculated as shown in the example in Fig. 8.4. In this example, a given temperature produced a kill curve with a D value of 2 minutes. A more heat-resistant microbe would have a longer D value under the same conditions. A more heat-sensitive microbe would have a shorter D value at the same temperature. In this way, it is possible to compare the heat sensitivity of different microbes, for example:

- *Campylobacter* has a D_{55} value of 1 minute. This means that it takes 1 minute to kill 90 per cent of *Campylobacter* at 55°C. It is relatively heat sensitive.
- By contrast, the D_{55} of spores of *Clostridium botulinum* would take so long to measure that the scientist doing the measuring would soon give up and go home! The spores are so heat resistant that even boiling at 100°C doesn't kill them. A temperature of 121°C is required to achieve a practical D value in food processing. The D_{121} for the spores is 0.2 minutes.

The presence of some ingredients, such as fat, protein and sugar, can have a protective effect on microbes during heating. An example of this is *Salmonella* in chocolate. The D value at 90°C for *Salmonella* is about 75 minutes in chocolate but less than a fraction of a second in milk.

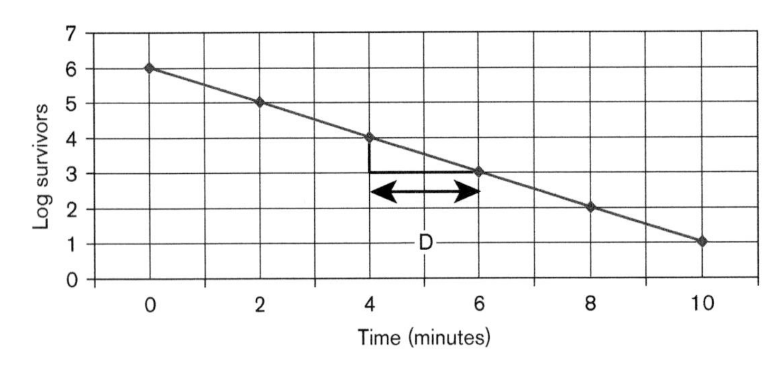

Figure 8.4 Calculating the D value for a microbe. At a given temperature, the death of a microbe can be monitored by counting the number of survivors and plotting the log of the numbers against time. The time needed to kill one log of the organism in this example is 2 minutes.

Canning

The temperature of boiling water (100°C) is sufficient to kill many bacteria, fungi and viruses but bacterial spores can survive boiling for many hours. A temperature of 115–121°C is needed to destroy these hardy structures. This requirement is achieved in the commercial process of canning. The technique is sometimes referred to as appertization after Nicolas Appert, a French confectioner who experimented with heating foods in sealed containers in the late eighteenth century. By the twentieth century, canning became a huge industry producing many familiar products such as baked beans, soups and tuna fish. Canning keeps foods preserved for at least a year and often several years for some products.

The time/temperature combinations used in commercial canning are governed by the properties of *Clostridium botulinum* (see Microbial CV for *Clostridium* in Chapter 7). The aim is to maximize the destruction, known as the '**botulinum cook**', of the bacterial spores produced by this organism. The tins of food are heated in containers known as retorts at 115–121°C for 25–100 minutes, depending on the acidity of the food. Since *C. botulinum* is fairly acid sensitive, less severe heat treatments are needed for acidic foods, such as tomato paste and fruit juices, while more severe heating is needed for low-acid foods, such as green beans and meats. Modern canning operations are now so carefully controlled that cases of botulism are quite rare. Quality control failures are occasionally manifested in the form of bent or leaking cans. Blowing of cans can sometimes occur due to the survival of spores from spoilage organisms such as *Bacillus stearothermophilus* (see Chapter 7, p. 92).

Pasteurization

Pasteurization is a milder form of heat treatment by comparison with canning. The shelf life of pasteurized foods is much shorter than that of canned foods but many of the flavours, textures and vitamins lost by the severe canning process are retained.

Pasteurization does not sterilize foods but it does reduce the number of microbes present drastically. The principles of pasteurization were first described by Louis Pasteur (Box 8.1) but in modern food processing, pasteurization is a set of carefully controlled steps undertaken on an industrial scale.

Like canning, pasteurization depends on the correct use of time/temperature combinations during heat treatment. An example of this is milk pasteurization. Raw milk is a precious commodity that spoils very quickly at room temperature and can contain enough pathogenic bacteria to make people ill. Boiling milk is an ancient way of killing the microbes in it but high temperatures also affect the taste and destroy some of the precious nutrients in milk.

Table 8.2 shows the three principal methods used for milk pasteurization. The older method of heating milk at 63°C for 30 minutes can be used for moderate volumes but for large quantities of milk the high temperature short time (HTST) and the ultra high temperature (UHT) treatments are now more common. In the

Box 8.1 Microbiology Hall of Fame: Louis Pasteur (1822–1895)

The modern method of pasteurization was named in honour of Louis Pasteur, one of the founding fathers of microbiology and a national hero in France.

Pasteur was a Professor at the University of Lille in the 1860s. In addition to his academic work, his remit was to work with local industries to help them solve practical problems. At that time, the wine industry was plagued by spoilage problems that made storage and shipping difficult. Pasteur examined some spoiled wines under the microscope and realized they were teeming with microorganisms. He then discovered that heating the wine at 55–60°C destroyed some of these spoilage organisms and preserved the wine for long periods of time. Unlike boiling, this treatment did not ruin the flavour of the wine or evaporate off the alcohol. This method was later adapted for milk, beer and many other liquid and semi-solid foodstuffs.

Pasteur was a prolific scientist. He went on to disprove the then popular but controversial theory that bacteria could arise from non-living matter by spontaneous generation. He proposed the germ theory of disease that explained the origins of diseases such as anthrax, cholera and tuberculosis. He also worked on the development of a vaccine for rabies. Pasteur's experiments laid the foundations for later work by Koch who proved beyond doubt that bacteria caused diseases (see Box 3.1).

industrial process, milk is pumped between metal plates (heat exchangers) or through pipes surrounded by hot water. This allows large volumes of milk to be processed quickly and ensures that heating is evenly applied throughout the liquid. In this way, cold pockets in which bacteria could 'hide' and escape the heat process are avoided. The heating step is followed by rapid cooling to 4°C.

Table 8.2 Time–temperature combinations used in the pasteurization of milk

Treatment	Holding temperature	Minimum time at holding temperature	Chill storage needed?	Typical shelf life
Ultra high temperature (UHT)	135–150°C	1–3 seconds	No	2–3 months (6–9 months if combined with sterile handling and packaging)
High temperature short time (HTST)	72°C	15–20 seconds	Yes	2–3 weeks
Low temperature pasteurization	63°C	30 minutes	Yes	2 weeks

In addition to milk, many other dairy and alcoholic beverages are routinely pasteurized. Examples include buttermilk, beer and wine. The small coffee-sized portions of milk and cream provided in hotels and restaurants are often prepared by UHT treatment. Semi-solid foods, such as yogurts, fruit purées, syrups and liquid eggs, are also suitable for pasteurization.

Cooking meat: how hot and how long?

If all meat and poultry were cooked thoroughly and eaten hot immediately after cooking, the number of cases of food poisoning would be greatly reduced. As it is, inadequate heating is one of the main factors responsible for many food-poisoning outbreaks.

The time and temperature required to kill pathogens in meat depend not only on the heat sensitivities of the microbes but also on the type of meat and the form that it is in. For example, as shown in Table 8.3, the D value for *Campylobacter jejuni* in lamb, which is more fatty than lean beef, is more than twice as long as in ground beef. Furthermore, it takes longer to kill organisms in solid pieces of meat than in liquids such as milk. The D value for *C. jejuni* is nearly three times as long in lamb as in skim milk at 50°C. At any specified temperature, it takes less time to destroy microbes in a smooth liquid such as milk or clear soup than in solid pieces of meat such as cubes, joints or steaks.

Table 8.3 D_{50} values for *Campylobacter jejuni* in milk, beef and lamb

Food	D_{50} value (minutes)
Skim milk	4.5
Lean ground beef	6.3
Lamb cubes	13.3

Guidelines for the safe cooking of meat have been developed in several countries. In the UK, the Government's Chief Medical Officer recommends that all meat products should be cooked to a minimum temperature of 70°C throughout the product for at least 2 minutes. Equivalent time/temperature combinations are also provided in the guidelines. These numbers were initially based on a reduction of at least 6 logs of *E. coli* O157 in beef burgers but the recommendations were subsequently broadened to encompass other heat-sensitive pathogens such as *Salmonella*, *Campylobacter* and *Listeria* in meat. In the USA, guidelines developed by the US Department of Agriculture (USDA) make a distinction between whole cuts of meat, ground meat and poultry meat. The guidelines for both countries are shown in Box 8.2.

Once cooked, how long and at what temperature can food be kept hot? Ideally, cooked meat, poultry and vegetable casseroles should be eaten immediately. If this is not possible, *cooked foods should be kept at or above 63°C (145°F) for no more*

Box 8.2 Heating recommendations for meat

Don't just guess these temperatures! Use a temperature probe or food thermometer, placed in the thickest part of the meat!

UK

Cook *all meat products to a minimum internal temperature of 70°C for at least 2 minutes*. The following equivalent temperature and time combinations can also be used:

- 60°C for 45 minutes;
- 65°C for 10 minutes;
- 70°C for 2 minutes;
- 75°C for 30 seconds;
- 80°C for 6 seconds.

Additional advice for chicken livers: cook to an internal temperature of 70°C or more for at least 3 minutes.

USA

Cook all *whole cuts of meat such as roasts, steaks and chops to a temperature of 63°C (145°F), then allow the meat to rest for 3 minutes* before carving or eating. The resting time is important because the food remains at the final temperature it reached in the oven, grill or other food source for up to 3 minutes. This recommendation applies to whole cuts of beef, veal, lamb and pork.

Ground beef, veal, lamb and pork should be cooked to a temperature of 72°C (160°F). These products do not require a rest time.

All poultry products including chicken and turkey should be cooked to 74°C (165°F).

than 2 hours. Alternatively, they must be cooled rapidly to below 5°C (41°F) and stored at this temperature until required when they should be reheated to 72°C (162°F) before eating.

A note about food for vulnerable groups

We have seen in Chapter 4 that some groups of people, such as young children, the elderly and the sick, are more vulnerable to infection by food-poisoning organisms and when they are infected, their symptoms are more likely to be severe. The proportion of vulnerable people in a typical foodservice establishment open to the general public can be as high as one in five. But in nurseries, hospitals, residential homes for the elderly and cancer hospices, the proportion of people in the vulnerable category may be as high as 100 per cent. Food professionals working in these establishments must be extra vigilant about food safety.

Vulnerable groups are particularly susceptible to infection by *Listeria monocytogenes* and verocytotoxin-producing *Escherichia coli* (VTEC) (Chapter 6), *Salmonella* (Chapter 5), and norovirus (Chapter 7). Therefore, the following foods should not be served to vulnerable people:

- Unpasteurized milk and fruit juices.
- Cheeses and yogurts made with unpasteurized milk; all blue-veined cheeses.
- Cold-smoked fish.
- Frankfurters (hot dogs) and lunchmeats, unless they have been heated to a temperature of at least 72°C or higher.
- Chilled deli salads, such as chicken salad, prawn mayonnaise, Waldorf salad.
- Lightly cooked eggs or foods containing raw egg (e.g. home-made mayonnaise, hollandaise, tiramisu, mousses made with raw eggs). Use pasteurized liquid egg instead.
- Raw or lightly cooked shellfish (e.g. oysters, mussels, clams, scallops), fish, and sprouts made from alfalfa, mung beans and fenugreek. These foods can be served if heated to a temperature of at least 72°C or higher.

Patients with certain cancers may need even more restrictive diets to avoid infection. Further advice and guidance from the American Cancer Society can be found in the weblink section at the end of the chapter. However, any modifications to the diets of severely ill people should be made only in consultation with clinical staff and an appropriately qualified dietitian.

Controlling microbial growth

Having killed off some of our undesirables as described above, we now turn to control methods designed to prevent the survivors from growing fast in foods.

There are many factors that influence microbial growth in foods but the three most important ones are:

- temperature;
- water;
- acidity (pH).

In this section, we explore ways in which each one of these factors can be manipulated to control microbes in food.

Temperature

Although some bacteria and fungi are capable of rapid growth at extreme temperatures, most foodborne pathogens have adapted to humans and warm-blooded animals and so have a limited growth range. Consequently, one of the most important ways of controlling microbes in foods is to maintain the temperature of the environment either above or below the ideal range for growth.

Each microbial species has an **optimum temperature** at which growth and multiplication are fastest. Below this temperature, the growth rate is slower, declining gradually until the *minimum temperature* is reached, below which no growth occurs. Similarly, above the optimum temperature, the growth rate decreases until the *maximum temperature* is reached, above which no growth occurs. These are sometimes referred to as **cardinal temperatures** and represent the growth range that characterizes each species. Fortunately, we do not have to remember the cardinal temperatures for every known foodborne pathogen as some generalizations are possible.

The optimum growth temperature for many bacteria that cause foodborne human diseases is, unsurprisingly, 37°C, the same as the body temperature of a healthy human. Bacteria such as *Salmonella*, VTEC and *Staphylococcus aureus* are adapted to living on humans and in soil and water in tropical and temperate climates. These bacteria grow best at moderate temperatures and so are known as **mesophiles** (ancient Greek for 'lovers of the middle'). Although the optimum growth range may vary slightly from species to species, as a general rule, temperatures between 28°C and 43°C provide ideal conditions for rapid growth of mesophiles. Growth below and above these temperatures still occurs but at a slower rate.

Many food-poisoning and spoilage bacteria and fungi do not grow well, or at all, at low temperatures and this is why chilling foods is such an effective method of microbial control. Chilling involves storing foods on melted ice at 0°C or refrigerating at temperatures just above freezing (–1°C to 5°C). Most foodborne pathogens cannot grow below 5°C, with the exception of *Listeria monocytogenes*, *Yersinia enterocolitica* and non-proteolytic *Clostridium botulinum*; these three species can grow very slowly at temperatures approaching 0°C.

It is important to remember that chilling does not kill microorganisms, it merely stops them from multiplying. Indeed, many microbes survive very well in chill temperatures. As soon as a chilled food is removed from the refrigerator, the temperature rises and the microbes start multiplying.

At the other end of the spectrum, the maximum growth temperature for many pathogenic bacteria is between 45°C and 50°C. Heating above 50°C gradually degrades the fine structure of the bacterial cell until complete kill is achieved, usually at 63°C and over.

From the above, it is evident that temperatures between *5°C and 63°C* represent the **temperature danger zone** for microbial growth. The longer a food is allowed to remain in this temperature zone, the more likely it is that microbial growth will occur. Many professional kitchens now use blast chillers designed to move food products through the temperature danger zone as quickly as possible. Figure 8.5 illustrates the key temperatures in microbial control.

Microbial growth can also be controlled by freezing. Most foods freeze at temperatures between –0.5°C and –3°C. During freezing, liquid water is made unavailable for microbial growth through the formation of ice crystals. Without liquid water, microbes cannot grow. Freezing and thawing can damage the fine structure of bacteria but is not an effective method of killing them. Indeed, microbiology laboratories use freezing as a method of preserving their culture collections for several years. Some reduction in numbers can be expected but many foodborne pathogens survive temperatures of –18°C or less for many years. For example, *Salmonella* has been isolated from ice cream and escargots (snails)

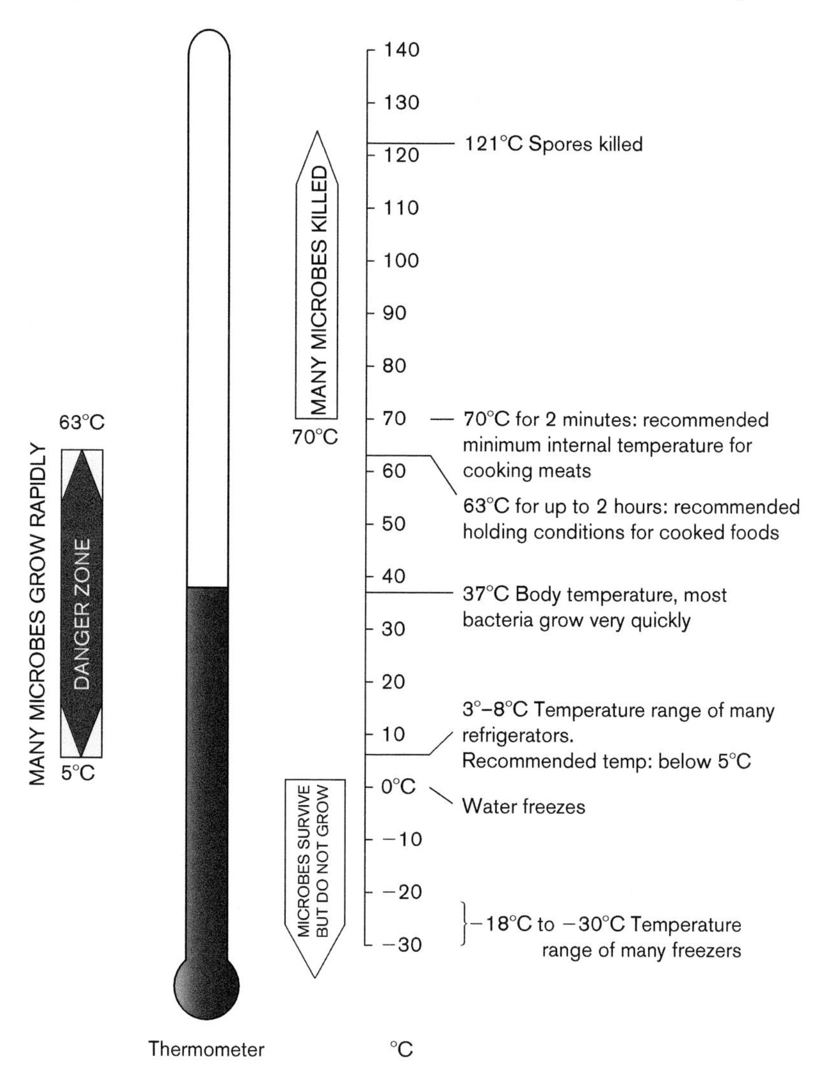

Figure 8.5 The importance of temperature in controlling foodborne microbes.

after 8 years in a freezer at –20°C. Bacterial spores and viruses are more resistant to freezing than vegetative cells and survive the process almost unscathed.

Some disease-causing parasites are sensitive to freezing and this can be exploited when preparing fish and shellfish intended to be eaten raw. Parasites known as nematodes (roundworms), cestodes (tapeworms) and trematodes (flukes) are not microorganisms but they form microscopic cysts or larvae in seafood. Examples of products that have been implicated in infection are ceviche (raw white fish marinated in lime juice and spices), sashimi (slices of raw fish) and sushi (pieces of raw fish with rice and other ingredients). As with cooking, the time/temperature combination and the type of seafood determine the efficacy of killing. The following conditions are recommended by the US Food and Drug Administration for fish that is no thicker than 15 cm:

- freeze and store at –4°F (–20°C) for 7 days;
- freeze at –31°F (–35°C) until solid, then store at this temperature for a further 15 hours;
- freeze at –31°F (–35°C) until solid, then store at –4°F (–20°C) for 24 hours.

These conditions are sufficient to kill parasites and are recommended for fish intended for raw consumption. It is arguable, however, whether fish that has been treated in this way can still justifiably be called 'fresh'.

Water

Water is essential for all life on Earth. But the mere presence of water in the environment does not guarantee that life can be sustained.

An environment can have large amounts of water present but it may be in a form that is not readily available for living organisms to use. For example, there is more than enough water in the Earth's oceans but that does not mean that we can meet our need for water by drinking seawater. Water can be tied up in ways that make it impossible for an organism to absorb it. We have seen in the previous section that freezing causes water to form ice crystals. Frozen water is solid and is not available for microbial growth. Similarly, water can become bound by chemicals to make it unavailable for growth. The way in which this happens is illustrated in Fig. 8.6.

The amount of water available for microbial growth is described as **water activity** (a_w). Pure water has a water activity of 1.0 and a completely dry material containing no water at all has a water activity of 0. Water activity is not the same as water content. For example, fresh meat has a water content of 75 per cent but a water activity of 0.98. This is because the bulk of the solids (protein and fat) present in meat are not soluble. Meat solids do not bind water and so there is plenty available for microbial growth to occur.

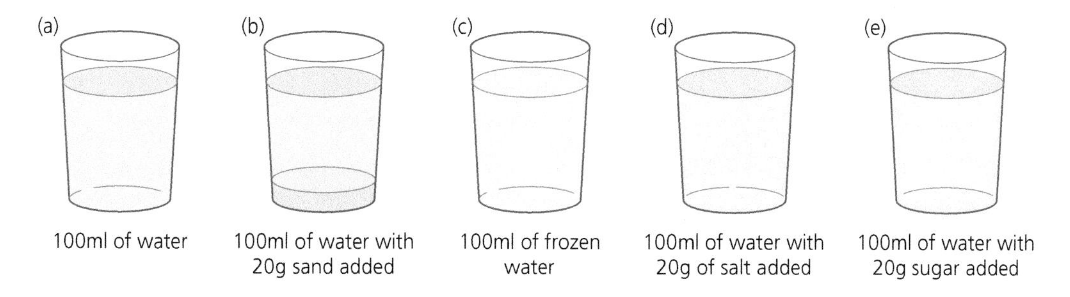

Figure 8.6 The availability of water for microbial growth. Beakers A and B: Water availability is the same in these beakers. Sand does not dissolve in or absorb water. Microbes can grow. Beaker C: Freezing solidifies water making it unavailable for growth. No organisms can grow. Beaker D and E: Salt and sugar dissolve in and bind water making less of it available for growth. Many microbes cannot grow. Adapted from Garbutt, J. (1997). *Essentials of Food Microbiology.* Arnold, London.

The ancient methods of food preservation by drying, salting or adding sugar work because the water is made unavailable for microorganisms to grow.

Each microbial species has a range of water activity for growth. Just like with optimum temperature, there is an optimum water activity for growth. For most foodborne microbes, the optimum water activity is very near the top end of the scale or 1.0. The minimum water activity for growth varies, depending on how well the organism is adapted to dry, salty or sugary conditions. As with temperature, generalizations are possible and these are illustrated in Fig. 8.7. Except for *Staphylococcus aureus* and *Bacillus cereus*, the majority of foodborne pathogens do not grow at water activities below 0.93 or in the presence of 48 per cent sucrose (sugar) or 10 per cent salt.

In general, bacteria are less tolerant of low water activities than yeasts and moulds. This is why foods such as jams, hard cheeses and cakes, which have a water activity of 0.90 or less, are usually spoiled by yeasts and moulds, not bacteria. The absolute limit for microbial growth is a_w 0.61. Dehydrated foods, such as dried soups and powdered milk, have water activities below this biological limit and are said to be microbiologically stable as long as they remain dry. For example, freeze-dried foods have a water activity of less than 0.1. For more examples of foods and their water activities, see Fig. 8.7.

Like refrigeration, reducing the water activity of a food by drying or adding salt or sugar prevents microbes from growing fast. The cells take longer to start growing, the growth rate is slow and the final number of cells produced is lower than would be possible under ideal conditions.

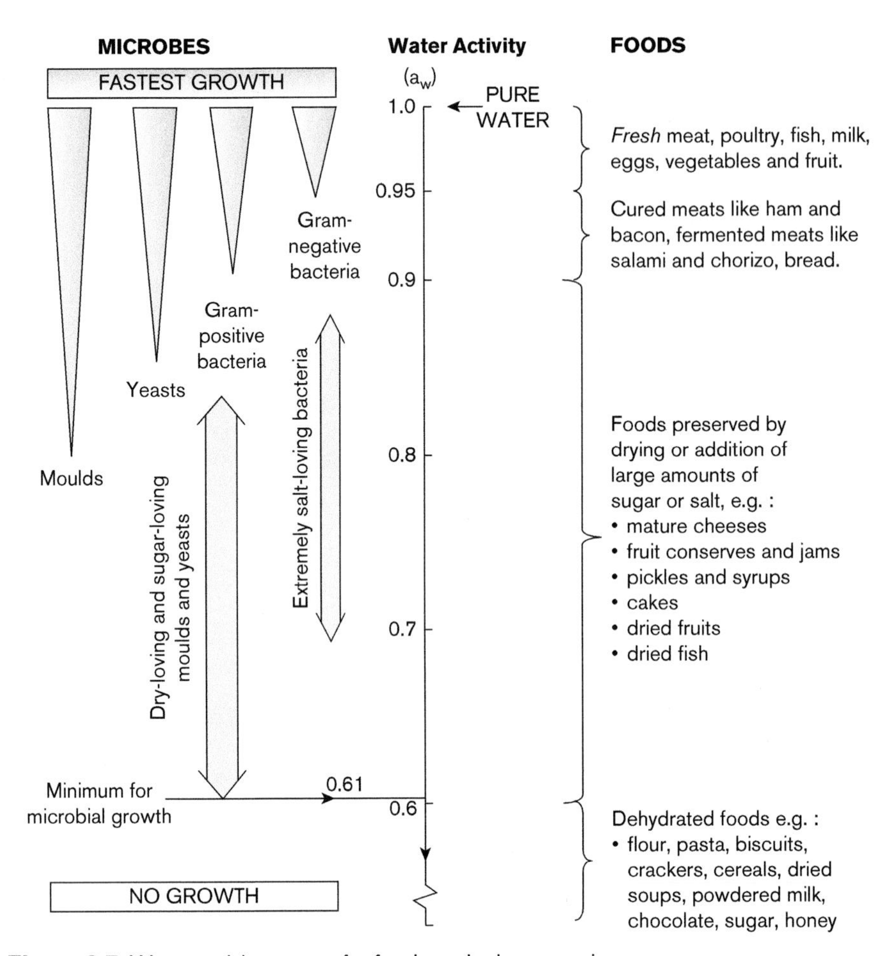

Figure 8.7 Water activity ranges for foods and microorganisms.

Like freezing, dehydration stops microbes from growing and reduces their numbers but does not kill the entire population that may be present. Indeed, just like freezing, microbiologists use freeze-drying as a method of preserving their culture collections for many years. Freeze-drying preserves microorganisms in a dormant state and is used by starter culture companies to store and ship their products to the fermentation industry in a light and convenient form. Bacterial spores survive drying even better than vegetative cells.

Acidity (pH)

In addition to temperature and water availability, there is a third factor that plays a very important role in microbial growth: the acidity (or alkalinity) of the environment. Acidity can be measured using a pH scale that ranges from 1 (very acidic) through 7 (neutral) to 14 (very alkaline). The pH scale reflects the concentration of ions in a solution or food. When the number of positively charged hydrogen ions (H^+) is equal to the number of negatively charged ions (OH^-), the pH is neutral. Put simply, pH is a measure of the acidity or alkalinity of a food.

All foods are either acidic or pH neutral. There are just two examples of alkaline foods. One of these, the familiar egg white, has a pH of 9. The second is an unusual Icelandic product called Hákari. This consists of shark meat that has been buried underground for up to 3 months and then dried for another 3–4 months. The degraded shark meat has a pH of 11 and contains high levels of pungent ammonia. Some consider Hákari a delicacy. Others would argue that it exists merely to demonstrate why alkaline foods are inedible.

As with temperature and water activity, each microbial species has a pH range for growth. The majority of foodborne microbes grow best at around neutral pH 7 and cease to grow above pH 9. It is at the acidic end of the scale that differences between organisms are more evident.

The pH ranges for both foods and microorganisms are illustrated in Fig. 8.8. The optimum pH for most food-poisoning bacteria is around 6.8 to 7.2 and the minimum around pH 4.1. Other bacteria such as those that are used to make fermented products are less acid-sensitive. For example, *Lactobacillus*, used in many dairy starter cultures to make yogurt and cheese, can grow at a pH as low as 3.8. The lactic acid produced by these harmless bacteria prevents the growth of food-poisoning bacteria and extends the shelf life of milk which would otherwise perish quickly.

As with water activity, yeasts and moulds can withstand more extreme pH conditions than bacteria. The optimum pH for many yeasts is around 4.5 and around 3.5 for moulds.

Like refrigeration and drying, reducing the pH of a food prevents microbes from growing fast. The cells take longer to start growing, the growth rate is slow and the final number of cells produced is lower than would be possible under ideal conditions. If the pH is reduced to well below the minimum for growth, many microorganisms gradually die off in acidic conditions, depending on the pH and the acid present. For example, *Salmonella* can survive in apple juice at pH 3.7 for more than 30 days but if the pH of the juice is 3.4 or less, the bacteria are killed off within 2 days. By contrast, *Salmonella* in pH-neutral egg droplets dried on surfaces has been reported to survive for more than 3 months.

Making foods more acidic by fermentation is an ancient method of preserving foods. Yogurt, cheese and salami are all examples of fermented products that have had their acidity reduced by the action of starter cultures. These cultures are often collectively referred to as lactic acid bacteria because of the main acid that they produce. However, other acids can also be used to adjust the pH of foods that are not fermented. For example, vinegar is added to sauces, mayonnaise and salad dressings. The active ingredient in vinegar is acetic acid.

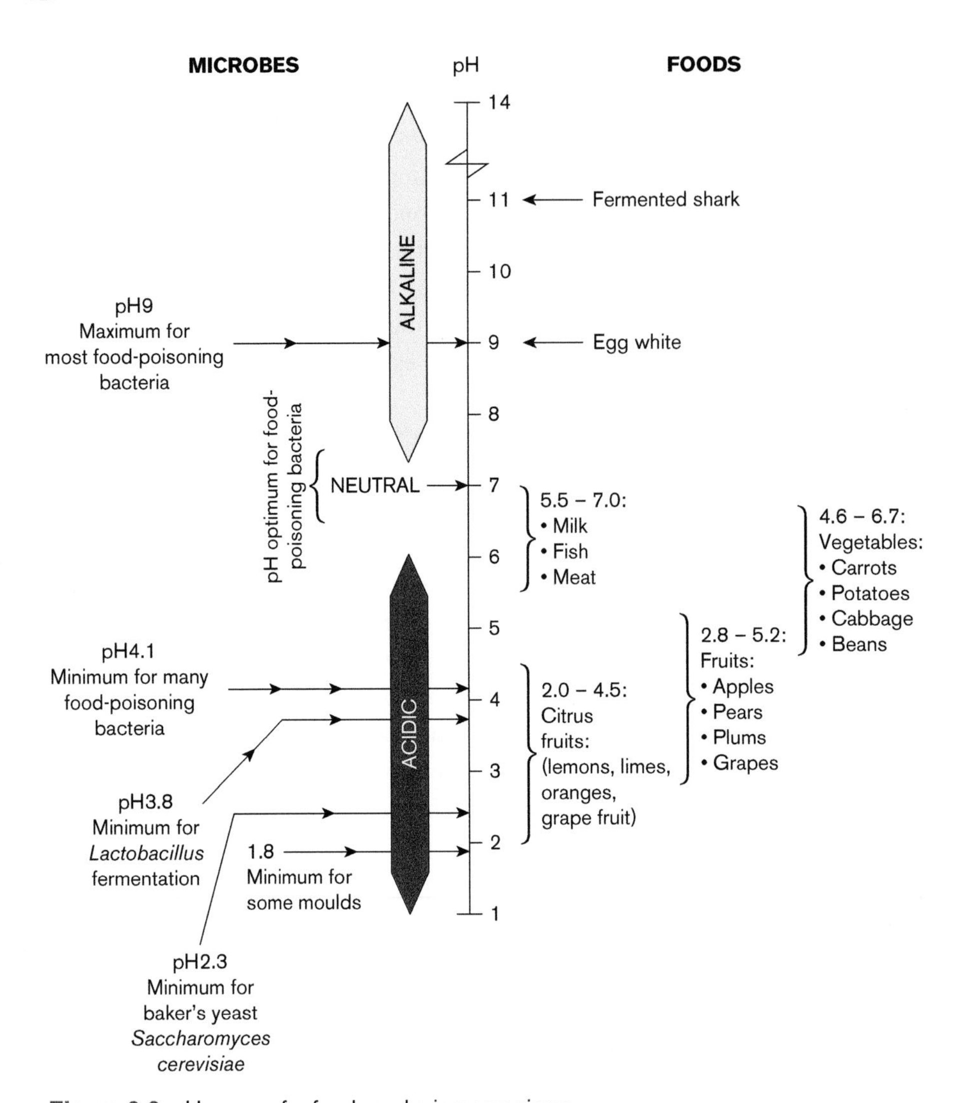

Figure 8.8 pH ranges for foods and microorganisms.

Not all acids are equally effective at killing or slowing down microbial growth. Table 8.4 shows some acids commonly used or found in foods and their respective strengths in terms of their action on microorganisms. The strength of acids is an important consideration when reformulating food products or changing recipes in a foodservice establishment. Replacing a strong acid with a weaker alternative reduces the shelf life of the product and increases the risk of survival of food-poisoning microbes. For example, as shown in Fig. 8.9, *Salmonella* dies off rapidly in mayonnaise made with vinegar (acetic acid) but survives and even grows in mayonnaise made with lemon juice (citric acid) at the same pH (4.4).

Table 8.4 Food acids and their properties

Acid	Found in	Strength
Hydrochloric	Added to soft drinks	Weakest
Phosphoric	Added to cola-style carbonated drinks	
Citric	Occurs naturally in lemon and lime juice Added to soft drinks, juices, jams and confectionery	
Malic	Occurs naturally in apples	
Lactic	Produced by lactic acid bacteria in many fermented foods (e.g. yogurt, cheese, salami, sauerkraut) Added to sauces, dressings and drinks	
Acetic	Produced in vinegar by *Acetobacter aceti* Added to sauces, dressings, mayonnaise, pickles, chutneys	
Propionic	Produced in Swiss cheese by propionibacteria starter culture Added to bakery goods and cheese spreads	Strongest

In the sections above, we have seen how temperature, water availability and acidity influence microbial inactivation and growth in foods. Each one of these factors could be used alone as a control measure in foods but in practice, it is more likely that two or more factors are combined. For example, pasteurization can usefully reduce the number of microbes present in raw milk but pasteurized milk can be kept even longer if combined with chill storage in a refrigerator. As another example, in traditional jam making, three control measures are used in combination: after *heating* the fruit to reduce the initial numbers of microbes present, the natural *acidity* of the fruit and the *low water activity* produced by the addition of sugar prevent many microbes from growing for several months.

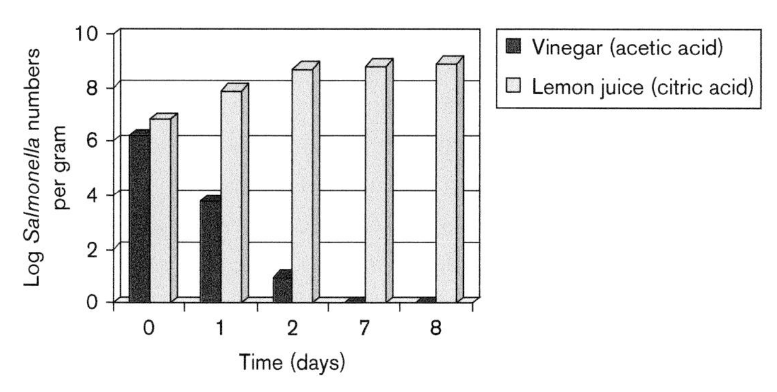

Figure 8.9 Salmonella dies off in mayonnaise (pH 4.4) made with vinegar but grows in mayonnaise made with lemon juice at the same pH. Data from: Lock, JL and Board, RG (1995). *Food Microbiology* **12**, 181–6.

In recent years, nutritional considerations and consumer demand for less heavily processed foods have led many food manufacturers to reduce the amounts of salt, sugar and synthetic preservatives in foods. These 'healthier' options would spoil much more quickly if an additional control method such as refrigeration wasn't used to prevent or slow down microbial growth. For example, low-sugar conserves and mild-cured bacon need refrigeration, unlike their traditional counterparts which can be stored at ambient temperatures.

Other methods of controlling microbial growth: preservatives and modified atmospheres

Food preservatives

Preservatives are added to foods in order to delay or stop growth of microorganisms that may spoil the food or render it unsafe for human consumption. Some preservatives can kill microbes but, in general, they are added in order to prevent growth. Preservatives are useful in controlling low levels of contamination and are not a substitute for good hygienic practices.

Many preservatives have been used since ancient times. For example, saltpetre, an impure form of crude salt, has been used to cure meat since the dawn of civilization. It was not until the 1920s that nitrate and nitrite were recognized as the active antibacterial agents in cured meat. The most important property of nitrite is its ability to stop growth of the spore former *Clostridium botulinum*. In addition to its antibacterial properties, nitrite is also responsible for the characteristic pink colour and flavour of cured meats such as bacon and ham.

Food preservatives, together with a host of other additives used to modify the colour, texture and flavour of foods, have acquired a somewhat tarnished image. In spite of strict regulations on the permitted levels and usage of food additives, some consumers regard any chemical addition to food as adulteration. So-called 'natural' methods of food preservation are seen as preferable to the use of synthetic additives, even though some of the most potent poisons on Earth are from natural sources. Ironically, when the European system of assigning 'E-numbers' to all legally permitted food additives was first introduced, it was intended to provide reassurance and guidance for their safe use. The E-numbers system has since been transformed in the minds of some consumers as a blacklist of food additives.

The most important food preservatives and their uses in the European Union are shown in Table 8.5. All permitted food preservatives, whether of natural or synthetic origin, as well as the acids shown in Table 8.4 have E-numbers.

Table 8.5 Examples of some commonly used food preservatives permitted in the European Union

E-numbers	Preservative	Source	Typical usage
E200–203	Sorbic acid and derivatives	Present naturally in berries of mountain ash; synthetic version used as additive	Low-fat spreads, fruit yogurts, processed cheese and cheese spreads, salad dressings
E210–219	Benzoic acid and derivatives	Present naturally in cranberries, greengage plums, tea and anise; synthetic version used as additive	Soft drinks, fruit products, bottled sauces
E220	Sulphur dioxide	Natural gas	Wine, cider, soft fruits prior to making into jam, dried fruits
E221–228	Sodium sulphite and derivatives	Synthetic	British fresh sausages
E234	Nisin	Produced naturally by fermentation	Processed cheese slices, clotted cream
E249–252	Nitrite, nitrate and derivatives	Natural salt	Cured meats such as bacon and ham
E290	Carbon dioxide	Natural gas	Carbonated drinks

Oxygen and other gases

The Earth's atmosphere or air contains approximately 20 per cent oxygen and 80 per cent nitrogen, together with a trace of carbon dioxide. Many bacteria, yeasts and moulds are perfectly adapted to this mixture of gases and grow prolifically in the presence of air.

Some microbes, including many spoilage moulds, require oxygen to produce cellular energy. Without air, they cannot grow. But others, including many foodborne bacteria and yeasts, are more versatile and can grow in either **aerobic** (presence of oxygen) or **anaerobic** (absence of oxygen) conditions. Many of the important food-poisoning bacteria such as *Salmonella*, VTEC and *Listeria monocytogenes* can grow in both aerobic and anaerobic conditions. When oxygen is present, more energy is produced and so growth is faster than under anaerobic conditions. A few bacteria, notably *Clostridium botulinum*, can grow only under strictly anaerobic conditions, that is, in the complete absence of oxygen.

Modified atmosphere packing

The composition of the atmosphere surrounding foodborne microbes can be controlled by modifying the gas mixture in the food pack. This is known as **modified atmosphere packing (MAP)** and it comes in three forms:

- vacuum packing (VP);
- gas flushing or modified atmosphere packing (MAP);
- controlled atmosphere (CA) storage.

All three forms of MAP are used in combination with refrigeration. Vacuum packing has become very popular in the foodservice industry, as it extends the shelf life of many foods and saves preparation time in the kitchen. In the retail sector, the combination of MAP with refrigeration has made it possible to develop a vast new range of chilled ready meals and ready-to-eat products that are sold directly to the consumer. The technology offers not only convenience but also a 'clean label' as no chemical preservatives are retained by the food once the packs are opened. The label on MAP foods simply reads: 'Packed in a protective atmosphere'. Like the food preservatives discussed above, MAP is useful in controlling low levels of contamination and is not a substitute for good hygiene.

At this point it would be timely to explain the meaning of shelf life. The **shelf life** of a food product is defined as:

> the period of time during which the food maintains its microbiological safety and sensory properties (flavour, texture, aroma) at specified storage conditions.

The shelf life of all foods is indicated on the packaging in the form of 'use by' and 'best before' dates. The two designations have very different meanings but are often confused by consumers and food professionals alike.

The **'use by' date** is about *safety* and often appears on foods with short shelf lives, such as fresh meat, chilled ready meals and prepared salads. Foods that have passed their 'use by' date should be discarded, as they could make someone ill. Storage instructions on such foods must be strictly followed as improper storage could make such foods hazardous before the expiry of the 'use by' date. For example, if chilled foods are stored in a faulty refrigerator, faster spoilage and food poisoning are more likely to occur. The shelf life of a chilled food can be extended beyond the 'use by' date by freezing it.

The **'best before' date** is about *quality* and is often used for foods with long shelf lives, such as canned, dried and frozen foods. If a packet of biscuits has passed its 'best before' date, this does not mean that eating it will make you ill. It simply means that the quality (flavour, aroma, colour, texture) will gradually deteriorate after that date. The biscuits will eventually become softer and the fats within them may become rancid, leading to off-flavours. Confusing the 'best before' date with the 'use by' date can lead to unnecessary waste of food that is still perfectly edible.

Some retailers use 'display until' and 'sell by' dates on their food packaging. These are instructions for shop staff, not consumers, and are intended to help with stock control.

Vacuum packing (VP) is the simplest form of MAP. A food product is placed in a plastic bag, the air is extracted using a vacuum packing machine until the packaging film collapses around the product and the bag is heat sealed. The choice of plastic packaging is important, as it needs to exclude oxygen but retain moisture. A range of plastic laminates is available, depending on the food to be packed.

VP is often used in the foodservice sector for bulk-packing of fresh meat and fresh-cut, ready-to-cook vegetables. Good-quality meat packed in a vacuum and chilled keeps up to five times longer than the same meat packed aerobically. Vacuum-packed fresh meat can sometimes look slightly off-putting as the meat protein myoglobin is purple without oxygen. However, this reaction is reversible and the red colour returns rapidly once the pack is opened and the meat is exposed to air. In the retail sector, VP is used extensively for cooked meats, sliced deli meats and smoked fish.

VP works by preventing growth of aerobic microbes. Some spoilage bacteria can grow in the absence of oxygen but they do so more slowly than would be the case under aerobic conditions. The main concern in VP is the potential for growth of non-proteolytic strains of *Clostridium botulinum*, particularly if the cold chain is not carefully controlled and temperatures creep above 3°C. At 10°C, *C. botulinum* can grow and produce toxin within a typical shelf life of 10 days. Consequently, all manufacturers of VP machinery are advised to include instructions regarding the risks of *C. botulinum* growth in VP foods. In addition, the Food Standards Agency in the UK has published guidelines regarding both VP and MAP foods as shown in Box 8.2.

Cuisine sous-vide (French for 'cooking under vacuum') is a variant of VP developed in the 1970s in France. This involves heating vacuum-packed foods at low temperatures and for a longer period of time than traditional cooking. The temperatures used are usually between 50°C and 65°C but can be as low as 40°C for fillets of fish such as cod and halibut. Since temperature control is crucial in this process, specially designed water baths are available for purchase by restaurants wishing to use the technique.

Cuisine sous-vide has been adopted enthusiastically by many top chefs because of the supposedly superior gustative properties of dishes cooked in this way. Meats are said to be more juicy and tender while vegetables retain more of their original flavour, aroma, texture and shape than traditionally cooked foods. However, the practice has a high element of risk because the cooking is done within the temperature danger zone (5–63°C) under anaerobic conditions and so may trigger germination of *C. botulinum* spores (see Chapter 7 for more on this organism). In addition, there is some evidence in the scientific literature that exposing pathogens such as *Salmonella* to mild heat 'stresses' equivalent to some of those used in *cuisine sous-vide* may render the organism more virulent (i.e. able to cause more severe illness).

Modified atmosphere packing (MAP) other than VP involves replacing the air normally surrounding a food with a gas mixture enriched with carbon dioxide. As shown in Table 8.5, carbon dioxide is used extensively in fizzy drinks to inhibit microbial growth. Not all microbes are equally sensitive to carbon dioxide. Moulds and many Gram-negative bacteria are very sensitive but some Gram-positive bacteria and several species of spoilage yeasts are more tolerant.

In MAP, food packs are flushed through with a gas mixture containing from 35 to 80 per cent carbon dioxide, depending on the product, with the remainder consisting of nitrogen and oxygen. During storage, the composition of the gas atmosphere changes due to respiration by microorganisms and foods, gas permeability of the plastic packaging and dissolution of carbon dioxide in the food to form carbonic acid. Large changes during storage can be reduced if the gas-to-product volume ratio is large. This is why meat joints are often sold in packs that seem excessively voluminous for the size of the product inside. Alternatively, oxygen scavengers may be used. These can be seen in packs of sliced deli meats where they often take the form of coin-sized sachets sealed to the inside of the lid and labelled 'Do not eat'.

Controlled atmospheres (CA) are used mainly for bulk storage of fruit and vegetables. In this way, it is possible to make seasonal produce such as apples and

Box 8.2 Safety recommendations for vacuum packed and modified atmosphere foods

Given the risks of *C. botulinum* growth in chilled vacuum packed (VP) and modified atmosphere packed (MAP) foods, the Food Standards Agency in the UK has issued a set of comprehensive guidelines as well as brief factsheets for all food handlers who make, re-pack or sell these products. The documents are available from the weblink section at the end of this chapter. Briefly, the main recommendations regarding the safety of VP/MAP foods are:

- A maximum 10-day shelf life is recommended for VP/MAP foods stored at 3–8°C if other controls are not used.
- For a shelf life of more than 10 days, in addition to chill temperatures, the following controls should be used, either on their own or in combination:
  - heat at 90°C for 10 minutes, ensuring that this temperature is reached in the centre of the thickest part of the food;
  - acidify food to pH 5 or less, ensuring that this pH is achieved uniformly;
  - add salt at a minimum of 3.5 per cent throughout all parts of the food;
  - reduce water activity to 0.97 in all components of the food;
  - other controlling factors may be used, including combinations with preservatives such as nitrite, but these must be shown to be safe using expert scientific advice.

pears available all year round. In this technique, the gas atmosphere in sealed tanks is maintained throughout storage by periodic flushing with 5–10 per cent carbon dioxide. This delays mould growth and also inhibits production of ethylene, a natural gas produced by the fruit to induce ripening.

The human factor: controlling microbes through personal hygiene, cleaning, preventing cross-contamination and workforce training

Personal hygiene

As mentioned in the Introduction to this book, humans don't help to keep food safe, they spread germs. This theme continues throughout the book and in Chapter 3, we've seen how any object touched by the human hand can become contaminated with microbes.

Humans carry many harmless as well as pathogenic organisms, including *Salmonella*, *Staphylococcus aureus* and norovirus (see Chapters 4–7) and spread them via their hands to surfaces and foods. Some examples are shown in Table 8.6.

Table 8.6 Examples of pathogens carried by humans

Source	Organism/s	Occurrence
Nose and throat	*Staphylococcus aureus*	30 per cent of the population are healthy carriers of *S. aureus* but up to 60 per cent can carry one or more other pathogens
Boils and cuts, skin infections	*Staphylococcus aureus*	10^8 bacteria/drop of pus from an infected cut
Faeces	*Salmonella*, *E. coli*, *Shigella*, Hepatitis, *Giardia lamblia* etc.	1 in 50 employees are highly infective and shed 10^9 organisms/g faeces
Faeces under fingernails	as above	10^7 organisms/g faeces if hands not washed after going to the toilet
Vomit	Norovirus	Just 10 viral particles are enough to cause disease

All food handlers should maintain the highest standards of personal cleanliness. Good hygiene starts at home. Regular baths or showers are necessary to clean all body parts and hair. Nails must be kept short and clean. The use of make-up should be discouraged as foundation creams encourage growth of microbes on facial skin. Cuts, spots and boils should be covered with a waterproof dressing, preferably coloured blue. Very few foods are blue unless coloured artificially and hence blue dressings are easier to find in a kitchen should they become dislodged during work.

Once at work, outdoor clothing should be removed and placed in a locker away from the food-preparation area. A clean uniform or chef's whites should be worn while handling food. Protective clothing designed for work should never, ever, be worn on public transport or in the car! Remove all watches and rings and leave them in the locker. Microbes thrive in the moist, warm environment under rings and if food particles get trapped in there too, they're in heaven! If hair is long, it should be tied up and covered with a protective hat. We all shed hair on a daily basis and loose hair must be prevented from dropping into food.

Check your own personal habits. Hair flicking, nail biting, ear scratching, spitting and zit picking are bad habits. Avoid touching your face, especially the nose, during food preparation. As we've seen in Chapter 7, the nose can be heavily colonized with *Staphylococcus aureus* and other bacteria, even in healthy people. If you need to sneeze or cough during food preparation, do so on the sleeved inside of your elbow, not in your hand. If you need to blow your nose, use disposable paper tissues, discard them in a suitable rubbish bin and wash your hands immediately. To help you remember this, think of the phrase used in a recent UK public health campaign: 'Catch it, Bin it, Kill it!' (for weblink, see section at end of chapter). In other words, catch your sneeze or cough in a tissue, bin the tissue and then wash your hands with soap and water.

Many countries have made smoking in the workplace illegal but these new laws have spurred some food handlers into developing new bad habits. For example, chefs in their full whites have been spotted smoking in filthy sheds or next to the rubbish bins at the back of their restaurants.

Apart from smoking, all hand-to-mouth contact should be avoided when preparing food. Don't chew gum, betel nuts, fingernails or pens and pencils. If you must taste the food during preparation, use a clean spoon every time.

Hand hygiene: the key to food safety

It is not possible to serve food safely without good hand-hygiene practices. Estimates vary but according to the London School of Hygiene and Tropical Medicine, thorough hand washing could reduce the global number of diarrhoeal cases by 50 per cent and save 1 million lives every year. Keeping hands clean is the single most important habit that all food handlers must learn.

In an observational study of the UK public, just 33 per cent of men and 60 per cent of women washed their hands after using the toilet. Of those who did wash their hands, men took 47 seconds and women 79 seconds to complete the task. An American study showed that 67 per cent of people washed their hands after using the lavatory but 95 per cent claimed that they did! So, next time you help yourself to peanuts from a bowl on a pub counter or at a party, think about all the other guests who may have dipped their unwashed hands into it before you came along! Detailed analysis of complimentary bowls of peanuts provided by one foodservice establishment in the UK revealed traces of urine from up to 25 individuals in each bowl.

Professional food-handler behaviour is often no better than that of the general public. In a survey of 1000 food handlers and their managers in small- to medium-sized catering businesses, nearly 40 per cent of staff admitted to not washing their hands after visiting the lavatory while at work. More than half did not wash their hands on arrival at work and before preparing food.

As shown time and again in food manufacturing, healthcare and domestic environments, good hand hygiene must become a habit in order to be effective. Bad habits are stronger than reason and undermine the work of the best trained professionals (Box 8.3).

Box 8.3 Quote: 'I'm a professional chef! Of course I wash my hands after using the toilet!'

Ask yourself:

- How often do you skip hand washing after using the toilet because you are in a hurry?
- How often do you give your fingertips a 'quick rinse' under the tap when you know you should have washed your hands with soap and water?
- How do you know that your hand washing is effective?
- How do you know that your team's hand-washing techniques are effective?

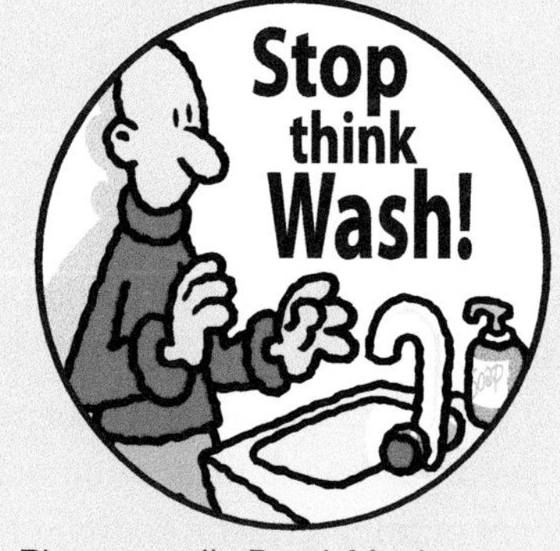

Picture credit: Derek Matthews

Next time you clean your hands, use the step-by-step guide in Fig. 8.10 to do it properly!

The simplest way of cleaning hands is by washing them with soap and water. The only effective way of learning how to wash your hands properly is to watch someone else doing it well and then copying the action in front of a trainer who can provide corrective advice. The second-best option is to watch a video clip of a hand-washing procedure. There are many videos of hand washing available on YouTube but they are not all reliable or appropriate for food handlers. Several weblinks to hand-washing videos prepared by public health authorities like the US Centers for Disease Control and Prevention (CDC) and the World Health Organization (WHO) can be found at the end of this chapter.

Box 8.4 Don't spread microbes. Wash your hands regularly throughout the day

Wash your hands regularly throughout the day but especially after:

- going to the toilet;
- entering a food room and before handling food or equipment;
- handling raw foods;
- handling money;
- combing hair;
- eating;
- smoking;
- coughing;
- blowing nose;
- disposing of rubbish;
- using chemicals.

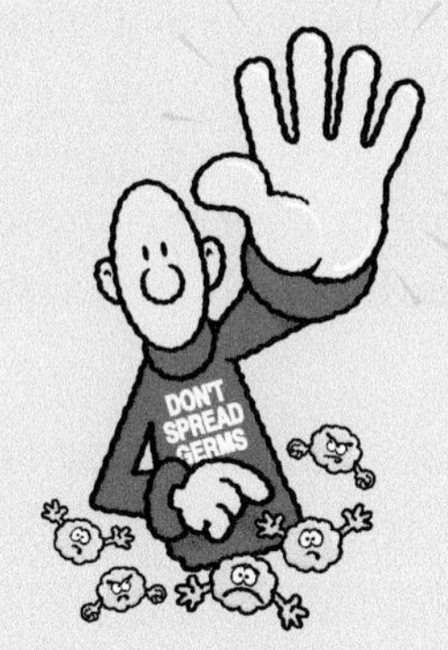

Picture credit: Derek Matthews

Figure 8.10 is a step-by-step guide to washing hands and using an alcohol-based handrub. The guide is available in 10 languages and can be downloaded from the WHO weblink at the end of the chapter.

A good hand-washing routine reduces the number of microbes on hands but does not eliminate them entirely. It is very important to dry the hands after washing because the microbes remaining on the hands spread much more easily from wet skin than dry skin. Disposable paper towels provide the most effective means of drying hands because they remove additional microbes from wet hands, they can be used to turn off the tap and they do not create aerosols (tiny droplets of water), which can spread microbes beyond the hand-washing area. Damp, dirty dishcloths should never be used to dry freshly washed hands. Drying hands on a dirty apron is even worse!

In many public washrooms, paper towels have been replaced by commercial air dryers but some older models are so slow that people often give up and leave before their hands are dry. More modern air dryers incorporate filtered air that is expelled through narrow slits creating high pressure 'air knives'. When hands are inserted between the air knives, moisture is stripped away in a controlled manner within just 10 seconds.

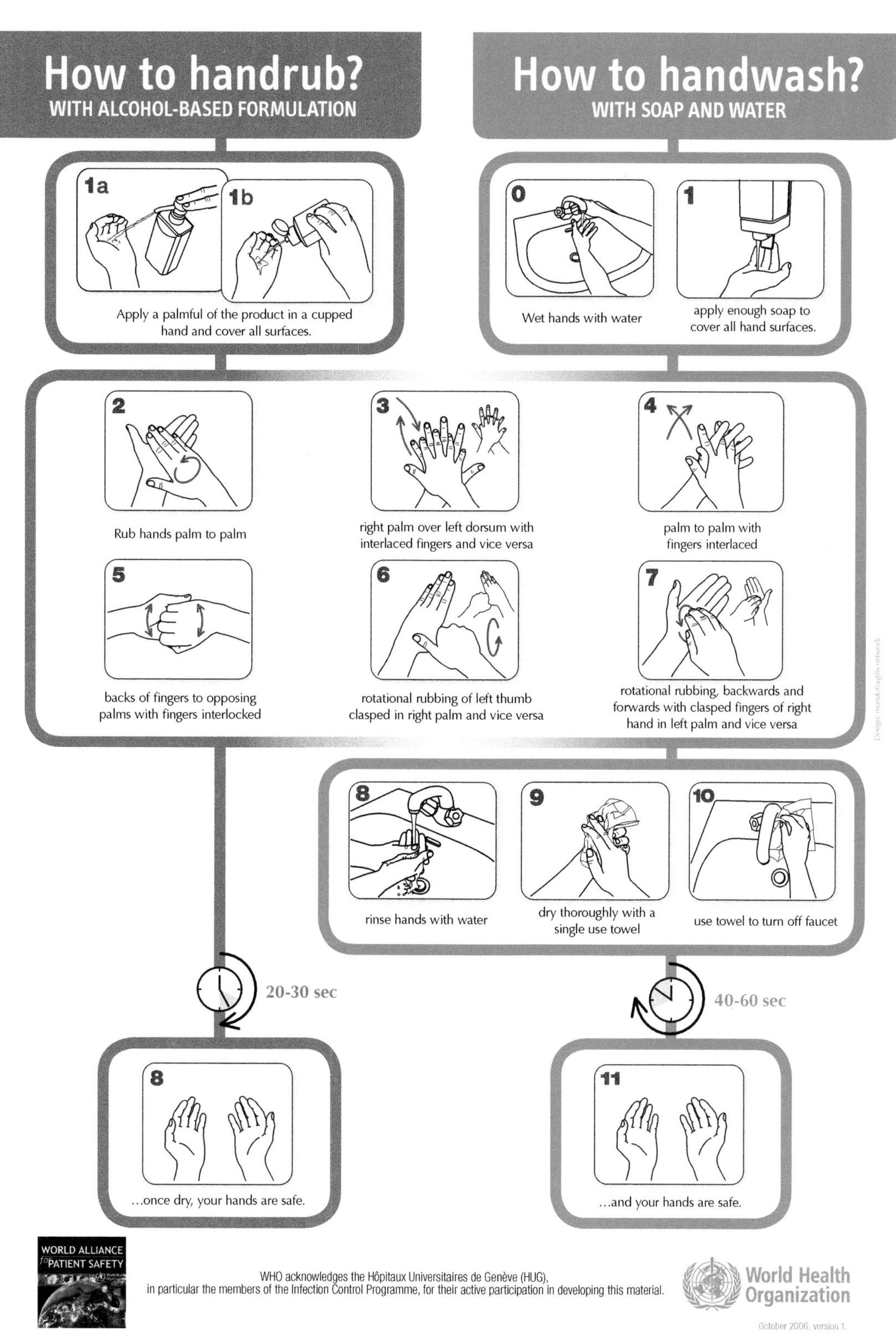

Figure 8.10 How to use handrub and wash hands with soap and water correctly. Courtesy of the World Health Organization (WHO).

WHAT DO YOU RECKON TO THIS ALCOHOL BASED HAND RUB?
HIC! I LOVE IT, I LOVE YOU...I LOVE HIC...EVERYONE!

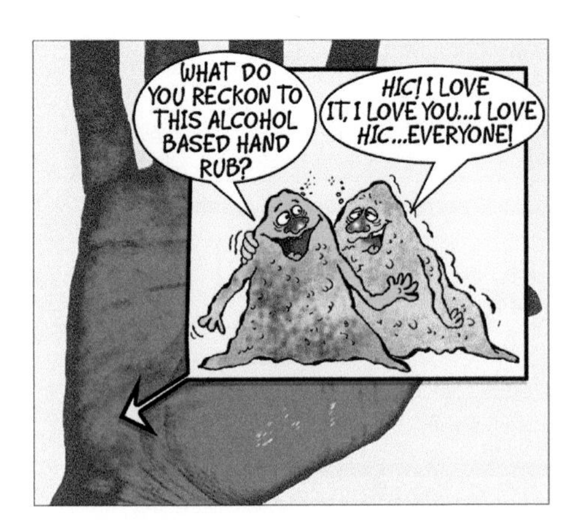

Figure 8.11 Some microorganisms are developing resistance to low levels of alcohol. Reprinted from Dixon, B (2008). There's the rub: Infection control that spreads infection. *The Lancet Infectious Diseases* **8** (2), 91, with permission from Elsevier.

When soap and water are not readily available, alcohol-based handrubs can be used to clean the hands. The main active ingredient in handrubs is alcohol (ethanol), often present at a level of 60 per cent. Other antimicrobial agents such as chlorhexidine may also be added together with a moisturizer that makes the handrub less irritating to skin than ordinary soap. Most handrubs are effective against bacteria but alcohol alone is not enough to inactivate norovirus and bacterial spores.

The use of handrubs was pioneered in the healthcare sector but the practice has become much more widespread. Wall-mounted handrub dispensers now feature not only in hospitals but also in food-preparation areas and even in office buildings. Pocket-sized handrub dispensers are also available from retailers for consumer use.

Some microorganisms are developing resistance to low levels of alcohol (Fig. 8.11). For example, *Acinetobacter baumannii*, a rival to methicillin-resistant *Staphylococcus aureus* (MRSA) and *Clostridium difficile* in the hospital-acquired infection race, not only tolerates the presence of 1 per cent ethanol but actually uses it to grow more prolifically.

Handrubs are effective, quick to apply and kinder to dry or inflamed skin than a soap-and-water routine. However, handrubs should not replace thorough hand washing, especially in heavily contaminated areas such as commercial kitchens, farms and lavatories. Soap and water should be the primary means of hand decontamination with handrubs used only as adjuncts to hand washing.

Like handrubs, disposable gloves should not be used as a replacement for hand washing but they can be helpful during preparation of ready-to-eat foods in a busy environment. For example, a food handler making sandwiches from scratch and handling money after each order is advised to use a fresh pair of disposable plastic gloves for each new order. Similarly, tongs and serving spoons should be used in preference to hands for plating out individual portions of food whenever possible.

Cleaning and disinfection

Cleaning and disinfection are very important for all food businesses in order to:

- prevent food poisoning;
- prevent contamination with foreign bodies (e.g. bone fragments, grit, fruit pips);
- prolong shelf life;
- discourage pests such as rodents, flies and ants;
- maintain good equipment performance;
- comply with the law.

Cleaning must be treated as an integral part of food preparation, not as an end-of-shift chore. It is easier to keep food-preparation areas clean if they have been designed hygienically in the first place. For example, dead spaces underneath kitchen cupboards that are difficult to reach with a mop should be avoided. However, very few of us are fortunate enough to have the opportunity to design a professional kitchen from scratch. Many professional food handlers have to put up with kitchen designs that are less than ideal in terms of food hygiene.

As we've seen in Chapter 2, microbes are invisible to the naked eye. Therefore, when trying to judge whether a surface is clean or not, our visual senses are useful only up to a point:

- If a surface is visually dirty, it is probably also microbiologically dirty.
- If a surface is visually clean, it is NOT necessarily microbiologically clean.

In any cleaning operation, the first step is to remove all large particles and food remnants sticking to surfaces. These not only protect microbes from the action of disinfectants but can also serve as sources of nutrients stimulating microbial growth. Detergents contain surface-active chemicals that help to dislodge soil particles, proteins and grease. Many detergents are alkaline, which dissolves fats and proteins. Some detergents are acidic and help to remove milkstone. Detergents are used in combination with physical methods such as scrubbing with brushes or pressure jets to dislodge firmly adhering soil.

In general, **detergents** do not kill microbes. Detergents remove microbes from surfaces making it easier to flush them down the drain and send them to the sewage farm for treatment by sanitation engineers. Therefore, a rinsing step is essential. Leaving dirty washing-up water to dry on dishes not only gives microbes another chance to re-attach themselves to the surface but may also taint foods with off-flavours.

Many microbes are inherently sticky and form biofilms (see Chapter 3) on surfaces that have not been cleaned and disinfected properly. Attached cells produce polysaccharide coatings that protect them from fluctuations in temperature and the killing action of disinfectants. Dead cells in the outer layers of biofilms often act as a protective barrier for cells that find themselves buried deeply within the biofilm matrix. Some types of kitchen equipment such as deli meat slicers are particularly susceptible to build-up of biofilms and must be cleaned regularly.

Disinfectants contain powerful antimicrobial chemicals but they don't work if visible dirt, food particles and grease are present. Food remnants reduce the efficacy of disinfectants by reacting with the active agent to neutralize it or by simply blocking access of the chemical to the microbial target. Pouring a disinfectant directly on to a soiled surface is a waste of money and time (Box 8.5). All visible soil must first be removed and residues must be rinsed off before a disinfectant is applied to a visually clean surface.

Chemical disinfectants contain a range of different antimicrobial agents that kill microorganisms:

- Oxidizing agents:
  - chlorine-based compounds (e.g. sodium hypochlorite): very effective but corrosive;
  - iodine-based compounds: effective but leave yellow taint;
  - peracetic acid and hydrogen peroxide: effective and used for fogging and disinfection of packing materials in the food industry.

Box 8.5 TV advert claims branded spray kitchen cleaner kills 99.9 per cent bacteria!

This may well be true, but:

- If there are 1000 bacteria on a kitchen top, killing 99.9 per cent removes 999 bacteria, leaving 1 organism on the surface.
- But, if there are 1 000 000 (or 10^6) bacteria to start with, killing 99.9 per cent removes 999 000 bacteria, leaving behind 1000 bacteria.
- If there are 1 000 000 000 (or 10^9) bacteria, killing 99.9 per cent removes 999 000 000 bacteria, leaving behind 1 000 000 (or 10^6) bacteria!

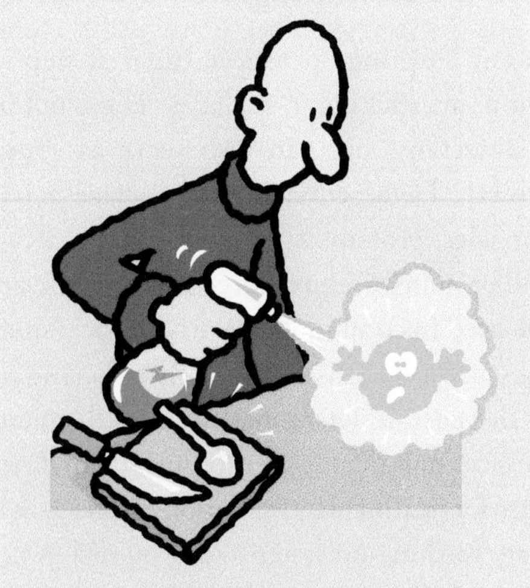

Picture credit: Derek Matthews

Conclusion

Although 99.9 per cent may look impressive, it won't work on a heavily soiled surface!

- Ammonia-based compounds (also known as quaternary ammonium compounds or QACs): non-corrosive but less effective.
- Triclosan, chlorhexidine: used in personal care products.

When choosing a chemical disinfectant, several considerations need to be made:

- What is the microbiological performance of the disinfectant? Is it active against vegetative bacteria only or does it also work against spores and viruses?
- Is performance affected by residual soil or water hardness?
- Is it hazardous to staff? What is the toxicity profile?
- Is tainting of foods likely if residues are left on dishes/equipment?
- What is the effect on equipment: is it corrosive, does it stain?
- What is the cost?

A disinfectant must be used at the correct concentration according to the manufacturer's instructions. Don't be tempted to dilute the disinfectant solution in order to save money. There is evidence in the scientific literature to suggest that some pathogens such as *Listeria monocytogenes* can become more virulent if exposed to sub-lethal concentrations of certain disinfectants. Many bacteria have molecular 'efflux pumps' (or 'vomit pumps' as they are affectionately known in the microbiology community), which enable them to bail out biocides that find their way into the cell. In this way, some bacteria survive low concentrations of disinfectants and other antimicrobial agents.

Like detergents, disinfectants must be rinsed off using clean drinking water after the recommended contact time is over.

Sanitizers have both cleaning and disinfecting properties in a single product but the two stages of cleaning followed by disinfection must nevertheless still be carried out.

In summary, the effectiveness of all cleaners, disinfectants and sanitizers depends on:

- chemical nature of the active ingredient;
- concentration used;
- time of exposure or contact time (in seconds, minutes or hours).

Materials impregnated with various antimicrobial agents have been used in health care for decades. For example, triclosan has been applied in fabrics used to make surgical gowns and gloves. More recently, such materials have also been introduced in the food industry and in consumer products. Triclosan has been incorporated into plastic chopping boards, food boxes, mixing bowls, brushes and dishcloths, bibs and potties for babies, toothbrushes and so on. Metals such as silver have been incorporated into refrigerator linings and plastic crates used to transport live poultry from farms to processing plants. These interventions reduce numbers of microbes on surfaces to a limited extent and do not replace the need for a thorough cleaning and scrubbing routine in a food-preparation environment. Furthermore, microbial resistance to both triclosan and silver has been reported.

How do you know if your kitchen really is clean? We have seen in Chapter 3 how swabbing and culturing microbes on agar can be used to assess the level of microbial contamination of surfaces. But this conventional microbiological technique is time consuming and expensive, requiring specialist equipment and microbiology laboratories. Most importantly, the results are not available immediately and a wait of 24–72 hours is often necessary. This is too slow to provide useful feedback about the efficacy of cleaning and sanitation.

Since the 1980s, a faster method based on measuring adenosine triphosphate (ATP) has been in development and has now gained acceptance in many food businesses. ATP is a molecule that exists in all plants, animals and bacteria as a source of energy. Its presence on a surface indicates that living cells are present. It is possible to detect ATP using an enzyme (biological catalyst) from the tail of the firefly to produce a yellow-green light. The amount of light can be measured to give a quantitative estimate of the amount of organic matter on a surface. The process takes just 20 seconds. Several manufacturers now produce hand-held meters and pre-treated swabs available to sample areas of 10 cm^2. The devices detect both microorganisms and food residues, and so are useful in hygiene monitoring before and after cleaning. This and other similar rapid methods have made it possible to take immediate corrective action if insufficient cleaning is detected.

Controlling cross-contamination

We have seen in Chapters 4 and 5 that cross-contamination is one of the main contributing causes of food-poisoning outbreaks (see pp. 57 and 71–72). *Salmonella* and *Campylobacter* are easily spread from raw chicken to ready-to-eat foods via hands, chopping boards and dishcloths (Table 5.2 and Fig. 5.2). Cross-contamination of ready-to-eat meat by VTEC originating from raw beef was identified as the key factor in two deadly outbreaks in the UK (see Chapter 6, p. 79). Therefore, any food business that handles both ready-to-eat foods and raw meat or fruit and vegetables that have been in contact with soil must implement the following three key control measures:

- strict separation of equipment and staff handling raw food from equipment and staff handling ready-to-eat food;
- effective cleaning and disinfection;
- effective personal hygiene and hand washing.

In large food-manufacturing operations, avoidance of cross-contamination can be built in at the design stage. The parts of the factory dealing with raw materials and cooked product can be separated by a wall with the cookers and ovens installed in between. These cookers can have doors on both sides with an entry on the raw side and an exit on the cooked side. The doors are designed in a way that they cannot be opened on both sides at the same time. The same principle can be applied to washing tanks for fruit and vegetables, with one side dedicated to incoming raw materials and the other to decontaminated or processed product. Members of staff are assigned to the raw side (high risk) or the cooked/processed side (low risk) of the factory and are not permitted to move freely between the two sides. Separate changing rooms for the two groups of staff can also be made available. Alternatively, strict changing room and personal hygiene procedures resembling those used in hospital operating theatres can also be implemented to minimize contamination of the high-risk areas.

Effective separation of raw and ready-to-eat foods can be achieved by providing a separate clean room or area with dedicated staff and equipment for the handling and storage of ready-to-eat foods only. Separate display facilities, refrigerators and freezers should be provided. If separate storage facilities are not possible, clean areas within mixed-use facilities should be clearly labelled and identifiable. Cleaning fluids, cloths and mops should also be kept separate.

Separate slicers, mincers and vacuum-packing machines should be used for raw and ready-to-eat foods. Delicatessen slicers are particularly vulnerable to heavy contamination and have been implicated in several outbreaks of *Listeria monocytogenes* in deli meats (see also Chapter 6). The risk of transfer must be minimized by regular cleaning. The US Food and Drug Administration (FDA) has produced a range of posters and flyers intended to assist front-line staff in maintaining slicer cleanliness. These materials are free of charge and are available in English and Spanish from the weblink section at the end of the chapter.

Staff must be instructed on the importance of cleaning their hands and changing their outer clothing (e.g. disposable aprons) when moving into the clean area from other working areas or when using shared equipment such as cash registers.

Separate chopping boards and utensils must be used for raw and ready-to-eat foods and they must be cleaned thoroughly between use. Many professional kitchens use colour-coded plastic chopping boards and signs reminding staff of their appropriate uses (Fig. 8.12). We have seen in Chapter 3 that microbes attach less readily to unused chopping boards made of plastic than those made of wood. However, once a plastic board has been scored with a knife, it is no better than wood in terms of providing a suitable surface for microbes to attach to. Nevertheless, plastic chopping boards are preferable in a professional kitchen because they can be colour-coded and washed at much higher water temperatures than wooden boards.

More information and advice on avoiding cross-contamination is available from the weblinks at the end of the chapter.

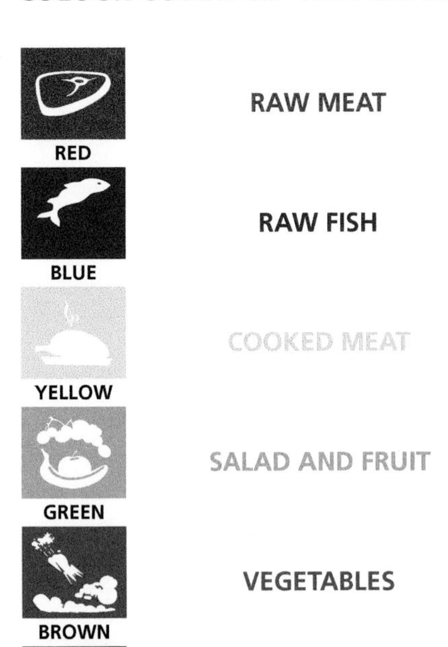

Figure 8.12 Plastic chopping boards can be colour-coded to indicate which food groups should be used on them.

Education and training of food handlers

Preparing foods safely is a skill based on knowledge. Therefore, food professionals need to be educated and trained before they can be expected to handle food safely.

Managers or owners of food businesses must ensure that they have a thorough knowledge of the management of food hygiene and that only trained food handlers are given the responsibility of preparing and serving food.

The level of education and training needed depends on the type of operation and job description of the food handler. In the UK, managers of food businesses are increasingly being educated at university level. Both 2-year foundation degrees and 3-year Bachelor's degrees in hospitality and culinary arts are awarded to hundreds of new graduates every year. Some of these go on to enrol on specialist Master's degrees in food control and food-safety management. Like the more science-based courses in nutrition, food technology and dietetics, these programmes invariably incorporate food safety, microbiology and hygiene in their curricula. Food safety is at the core of these subjects and is prescribed in subject benchmark statements published by the Quality Assurance Agency (for weblink, see end of chapter).

Many food handlers do not attend universities or hotelier schools but need specific training and education appropriate for the nature of their job. In the UK, there are several nationally recognized food-hygiene and safety courses and qualifications available. Some examples of these, provided by the Chartered Institute for Environmental Health (CIEH) are shown in Table 8.7. Other organizations such as the Royal Society for the Protection of Health (RSPH) as well as a multitude of public and private providers offer similar courses. Weblinks to some of these can be found at the end of the chapter.

Table 8.7 Nationally recognized food-safety courses and qualifications offered by the Chartered Institute for Environmental Health (CIEH) in the UK

Level	Qualification/award	Intended for	Duration and assessment
1	Food-Safety Awareness in Catering Induction into Food Safety for Manufacturing Food-Safety Awareness for Retail	New employees with no prior food-safety knowledge or training; employees handling low-risk or wrapped foods; front-of-house staff such as waiting or check-out staff; back-of-house employees such as kitchen porters or warehouse staff	Half day Multiple-choice exam
2	Food Safety in Catering Food Safety for Manufacturing Food Safety for Retail (Formerly known as the Basic Food Hygiene Certificate)	Anyone working with food in pubs, hotels, restaurants, retail, manufacturing, hospitals, care homes, schools and prisons	1 day Multiple-choice exam Course also available by e-learning
2	Refresher Food Safety	All who have taken the Level 2 Food Safety course three or more years earlier	Remote completion of workbook plus 1-hour discussion; or 3-hour training session
2	Cleaning in Food Premises	In-house and contract cleaners of food premises	1 day Multiple-choice exam
3	Supervising Food Safety in Catering Food Safety Supervision for Manufacturing Food Safety Supervision for Retail (Formerly known as the Intermediate Food Hygiene Certificate)	Managers and supervisors in small, medium and large food businesses	3 days Multiple-choice exam
4	Managing Food Safety in Catering Food Safety Management for Manufacturing (Formerly known as the Advanced Food Hygiene Certificate)	Production managers, trainers, owners, supervisors, auditors	5 days Assignment and exam

In recognition of the link between poor staff training and food poisoning, many other industrialized countries have developed training and certification schemes for food handlers. The courses give food handlers a basic understanding of hygiene, why it is necessary and how to achieve it. The core curriculum for a basic hygiene course often includes:

- Microorganisms as main cause of food spoilage and food poisoning.
- Characteristics of the main types of foodborne diseases.
- Control of microbial growth, survival and contamination.
- Personal hygiene DOs and DON'Ts.
- Principles of handling and storage (temperature monitoring, stock rotation and avoidance of cross-contamination).
- Correct cleaning.
- Common pests and their control.
- Introduction to food law.

Although managers are legally responsible for ensuring that employees have the necessary skills in food hygiene, these skills need not be obtained by attending formal training courses. They can also be obtained by self-study, relevant prior experience or on-the-job training. There is currently no legal requirement for all food handlers to attend an accredited training course in food safety. The absence of a licensing scheme based on evidence of knowledge is a weakness in current food-safety assurance. Whether or not mandatory training and licensing would help to reduce the number of food-poisoning cases has been the subject of much debate among professionals and the public.

Staff training is necessary but is not sufficient to achieve safer food-handling practices. Management buy-in and drive are also important. Following training, frequent reminders are necessary to reinforce food-safety messages. To this end, there are many resources available in the form of posters and leaflets that can be displayed in strategic areas of the workplace.

For example, the WHO introduced a 'Five keys to safer foods' poster in 2001. Reproduced in Fig. 8.13, the poster is now available, free-of-charge, in the six official WHO languages (Arabic, Chinese, English, French, Russian and Spanish) as well as in another 50 world languages, such as Creole Haiti, Zulu, Tswana and Serbian (printed in both the Latin and Cyrillic alphabets). The poster has been used in educational projects all over the world. The weblink for the poster is at the end of this chapter. Another example of a food-hygiene message is shown in Box 8.6.

Compliance with hand hygiene is often difficult to achieve. Knowledge of the need to wash hands after using the toilet is important but is not sufficient to overcome bad habits. Reminders on posters such as the example shown in Fig. 8.10 are necessary. A more drastic measure such as automatic locking of lavatory doors

Five keys to safer food

Keep clean

- Wash your hands before handling food and often during food preparation
- Wash your hands after going to the toilet
- Wash and sanitize all surfaces and equipment used for food preparation
- Protect kitchen areas and food from insects, pests and other animals

Why?

While most microorganisms do not cause disease, dangerous microorganisms are widely found in soil, water, animals and people. These microorganisms are carried on hands, wiping cloths and utensils, especially cutting boards and the slightest contact can transfer them to food and cause foodborne diseases.

Separate raw and cooked

- Separate raw meat, poultry and seafood from other foods
- Use separate equipment and utensils such as knives and cutting boards for handling raw foods
- Store food in containers to avoid contact between raw and prepared foods

Why?

Raw food, especially meat, poultry and seafood, and their juices, can contain dangerous microorganisms which may be transferred onto other foods during food preparation and storage.

Cook thoroughly

70°C

- Cook food thoroughly, especially meat, poultry, eggs and seafood
- Bring foods like soups and stews to boiling to make sure that they have reached 70°C. For meat and poultry, make sure that juices are clear, not pink. Ideally, use a thermometer
- Reheat cooked food thoroughly

Why?

Proper cooking kills almost all dangerous microorganisms. Studies have shown that cooking food to a temperature of 70°C can help ensure it is safe for consumption. Foods that require special attention include minced meats, rolled roasts, large joints of meat and whole poultry.

Keep food at safe temperatures

Danger zone!

60°C

5°C

- Do not leave cooked food at room temperature for more than 2 hours
- Refrigerate promptly all cooked and perishable food (preferably below 5°C)
- Keep cooked food piping hot (more than 60°C) prior to serving
- Do not store food too long even in the refrigerator
- Do not thaw frozen food at room temperature

Why?

Microorganisms can multiply very quickly if food is stored at room temperature. By holding at temperatures below 5°C or above 60°C, the growth of microorganisms is slowed down or stopped. Some dangerous microorganisms still grow below 5°C.

Use safe water and raw materials

- Use safe water or treat it to make it safe
- Select fresh and wholesome foods
- Choose foods processed for safety, such as pasteurized milk
- Wash fruits and vegetables, especially if eaten raw
- Do not use food beyond its expiry date

Why?

Raw materials, including water and ice, may be contaminated with dangerous microorganisms and chemicals. Toxic chemicals may be formed in damaged and mouldy foods. Care in selection of raw materials and simple measures such as washing and peeling may reduce the risk.

Food Safety
World Health Organization

Knowledge = Prevention

WHO/SDE/PHE/FOS/01.1
Distribution: General
Original: English

Figure 8.13 The World Health Organization (WHO) poster 'Five keys to safer food'. Available from: http://www.who.int/foodsafety/consumer/5keys/en/index. html

Box 8.6 The four Cs of food safety

The four Cs of food safety:

Cooking

Chilling

Cleaning

Avoiding **C**ross-contamination

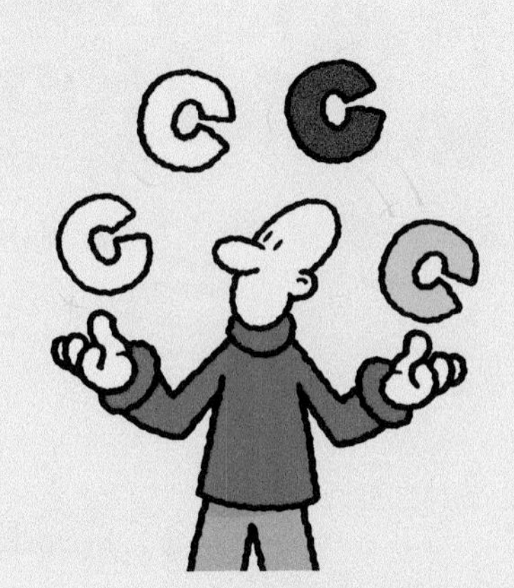

Picture credit: Derek Matthews

unless the hand-washing basin has been used has reportedly been very effective in persuading people to wash their hands in a hotel restaurant in France.

Hand-hygiene posters may appeal to fear. For example, a poster showing an image of a grave and stating 'Don't have a customer's death on your hands – wash them now!' can sometimes sell the message of hand hygiene more effectively by reminding people that food poisoning is more than just 'a bit of a stomach-ache'.

Conclusion

We have seen in this chapter that a plethora of control measures is available to ensure that our food supply is as safe as possible. When such measures fail, the consequences can be very serious, resulting in sickness and death by food poisoning, customer complaints, wasted food due to excessive spoilage, adverse publicity for the food business, fines, closure and loss of jobs and livelihoods. In the next two chapters, we discuss two more weapons available to us in the battle against foodborne diseases: prevention by Hazard Analysis Critical Control Point (HACCP) and the law.

Chapter 8 Quiz

1. A chef is seen smoking on the pavement in front of a restaurant. He is wearing protective overalls, an apron and blue plastic gloves. What is wrong with this and why?

Chapter 8 Exercise 1

Microbial growth depends primarily on temperature, acidity (pH) and water activity (a_w). Other factors may also play a role (e.g. food preservatives, composition of the gas atmosphere, etc.).

In the following table, list all the microbial control measures used in products made from the named food groups. The first line of each food group is already completed as an example. If the product is unfamiliar, go to the nearest supermarket and start reading some labels!

Microbial control measures **Milk and milk products**	
Pasteurized milk	Heating to pasteurization temperatures (e.g. 72°C for 15 seconds) Chill storage below 5°C
UHT milk	
Sweetened condensed milk in a can	
Dried milk powder	
Cream	
Yogurt	
Cheese	
Meat and meat products	
VP fresh beef joint for catering trade	Lack of oxygen Chill storage below 5°C
MA packed fresh pork roast in retailer's pack	
Canned corned beef	
Frozen minced beef	
Pâté	

continued ➢

Sweetcure bacon rashers	
Salami slices in retail pack	
Fish and fish products	
Frozen, oven-ready breaded cod fillets	Freezing arrests microbial growth, water is solid
Canned tuna	
Bacalao (dried fish)	
Rollmops (marinated herring)	
Thai fish sauce	
VP, cold-smoked salmon	
Sushi	
Wheat and wheat products: from noodles to strudels!	
Madeira cake	Heating during baking Low a_w
Sliced sourdough bread	
Chocolate éclair	
Prawn and mayonnaise vol-au-vents	
Spaghetti	
Fresh tortellini filled with spinach and ricotta in MAP	
Wheat flour	

Chapter 8 Exercise 2

Your line manager has tasked you with developing a new chocolate mousse recipe to be launched at a gala dinner for 300 people. You have decided to test two different methods of preparing the mousse. One method, involving a heating step, is safer but more time consuming. You also suspect that chill-storing so many mousses may be problematic for the business you work in. You decide to send samples of the finished mousse to a laboratory for analysis so that you can make an informed decision and advise your manager accordingly.

Your recipe contains the following basic ingredients:

- 110 g pasteurized milk;
- 140 g fresh egg yolk;
- 90 g sugar;
- 600 g couverture (dark chocolate containing at least 53 per cent cocoa fat);
- 800 g pasteurized whipping cream.

You prepare the mousse as follows:

Method 1: Heat-treated chocolate mousse	Method 2: Chocolate mousse with no heat treatment
1. Whisk the milk, egg yolks and sugar. Heat the mixture to 72°C while whisking. Measure the exact temperature of the mixture with a thermometer. Allow to cool to 30°C. This is known as the Anglaise method. 2. Whip the cream separately. 3. Melt the chocolate using the microwave oven. Use 30-second bursts with stirring in-between to avoid burning. 4. Fold the melted chocolate into the egg mixture, then fold in the whipped cream. 5. Label three lidded pots with the following: • Day 0 (day of preparation) • 3 days in fridge • Overnight in cool larder. 6. Divide the chocolate mousse into the pots in roughly equal amounts. 7. Send all mousses to the laboratory for analysis using express or same-day delivery.	1. Whisk the milk, egg yolks and sugar until light and fluffy. 2. Whip the cream separately. 3. Melt the chocolate using the microwave oven. Use 30-second bursts with stirring in-between to avoid burning. 4. Fold the melted chocolate into the egg mixture, then fold in the whipped cream. 5. Label three lidded pots with the following: • Day 0 (day of preparation) • 3 days in fridge • Overnight in cool larder. 6. Divide the chocolate mousse into the pots in roughly equal amounts. 7. Send all mousses to the laboratory for analysis using express or same-day delivery.

continued ➢

One week later: you receive the report from the laboratory and it shows the following:

	Method 1: Heat-treated		Method 2: No heat treatment	
	Total bacterial count per gram	Salmonella detected in 25 g	Total bacterial count per gram	Salmonella detected in 25 g
Day of preparation (Day 0)	470	Negative	7200	Positive
3 days in fridge	260	Negative	6500	Positive
Overnight in cool larder	4200	Negative	95000	Positive

Question A: Which ingredients in the mousse are high risk in terms of food safety and what was the most likely source of the *Salmonella*? Explain your answer.

Question B: Was the cool larder adequate for storing mousse? Explain your answer.

Question C: What recommendations would you make to your line manager regarding the preparation and storage of the mousses for the gala dinner? Could some of the ingredients be replaced with safer alternatives?

Chapter 8 Exercise 3

What cleaning and disinfection products have you seen used in food-preparation areas at your workplace or domestic kitchen? Write down some of the names of the products and look at the ingredients list on the labels. Which of the ingredients do you think might be responsible for killing microbes? Discuss your answers with your classmates.

Further reading

Pawsey, RK (2002). *Case studies in food microbiology for food safety and quality.* Royal Society of Chemistry, London.

Weblinks

FOOD-INFO is a multilingual food information site. It offers a wealth of information on E-numbers, food additives and food safety, as well as a food

dictionary in 20 world languages, including several non-European ones. Established in 1999, this website is kept up to date by a European collaborative team led by Wageningen University, Netherlands. Visit the site at:
http://www. food-info. net/

For a comprehensive list of pH values of dairy products, meat, fish, eggs, vegetables, fruits, bakery products and beverages, see the Appendix to the US FDA *Bad bug book*, available from:
http://www. fda. gov/Food/FoodSafety/FoodborneIllness/FoodborneIllnessFoodbornePathogensNaturalToxins/BadBugBook/ucm122561.htm

Food Standards Agency (2008). *Guidance on the safety and shelf-life of vacuum and modified atmosphere packed chilled foods with respect to non-proteolytic* Clostridium botulinum. Available from:
http://www. food. gov. uk/foodindustry/guidancenotes/foodguid/vacpac
and in pdf form from:
http://www. food. gov. uk/multimedia/pdfs/publication/vacpacguide. pdf
http://www. food. gov. uk/multimedia/pdfs/publication/vacpack0708.pdf

UK Department of Health. *Catch it, Bin it, Kill it. Respiratory and hand hygiene campaign 2007–2011.* Guidance, posters and radio announcements available from:
http://www. dh. gov. uk/en/Publicationsandstatistics/Publications/PublicationsPolicyAndGuidance/DH_123234

Guidance for food businesses on controlling cross-contamination, a question and answer leaflet and a factsheet are available from:
http://www. food. gov. uk/foodindustry/guidancenotes/hygguid/ecoliguide

The WHO '*Five keys to safer food*' poster is available in 56 languages from:
http://www. who. int/foodsafety/consumer/5keys/en/index. html

Materials on cleaning and maintaining commercial deli slicers are available in English and Spanish from:
http://www. fda. gov/Food/FoodSafety/RetailFoodProtection/IndustryandRegulatoryAssistanceandTrainingResources/ucm240554.htm

Link for American Cancer Society advice on food safety for people with cancer:
http://www. cancer. org/acs/groups/cid/documents/webcontent/002871-pdf. pdf

Hand hygiene

Put your hands together. Video clip, running time 3:38 minutes, first released in 2008 by CDC is available from:
http://www. cdc. gov/cdctv/handstogether/

Save lives: clean your hands. WHO's global annual campaign is available from: **http://www. who. int/gpsc/5may/en/**

http:www. handhygiene. org/ includes a link to a hand hygiene video from the University of Geneva

The step-by-step guide to using handrubs and washing hands (reproduced in Fig. 8.10) is available in 10 languages and can be downloaded from: **http://www. who. int/gpsc/tools/GPSC-HandRub-Wash. pdf**

Training and education in food safety and hygiene

Subject benchmark statements for honours degrees in the UK are available from: **http://www. qaa. ac. uk/AssuringStandardsAndQuality/subject-guidance/ Pages/Subject-benchmark-statements. aspx**

Courses developed by the Chartered Institute of Environmental Health are available from: **http:www. cieh. org/training/food_safety. html**

Many other organizations also provide training in food safety and hygiene, for example:
The Royal Society for Public Health
http://www. rsph. org. uk/en/qualifications/qualifications/qualifications. cfm
Reading Scientific Services Ltd
http://www. rssl. com/services/foodanalysis/foodtraining/ inhousefoodtrainingcourses/pages/inhousetrainingcourses. aspx
Leatherhead Food Research
http://www. leatherheadfood. com/online-training-courses
Campden BRI
http://www. campden. co. uk/food-safety-courses. htm

Section III: Desserts and Cheese

'From whence I conclude that the Vinegar with which I washt my Teeth, kill'd only those Animals which were on the outside of the scurf, but did not pass thro the whole substance of it.'

Antony van Leeuwenhoek, amateur microscopist and discoverer of microorganisms, 1684

9

Prevention is better than cure: HACCP

Before the 1970s, controlling the microbiological safety and quality of food was based largely on end-product testing and inspection. This was not a satisfactory system. The only way of assuring a safe food supply was to test 100 per cent of the food, an approach that would have left nothing to eat! Furthermore, as we have seen in Chapters 3 and 4, many conventional techniques for detecting microbes are retrospective and take too long to produce results. A more proactive, preventative system was required to assure food safety.

The Hazard Analysis and Critical Control Point (HACCP) system was pioneered by the Pillsbury Company working with NASA on the American manned space programme. It was essential to ensure that astronauts did not become ill with food poisoning during their space missions. Bouts of diarrhoea or vomiting in a weightless space station cabin or inside a space suit were to be avoided at all costs. The HACCP system of anticipating what could possibly go wrong at each step of the operation was born.

The HACCP concept is essentially a detailed analysis of each individual processing step, what could go wrong at every step and what can be done to prevent and correct every anticipated failure. It is a systematic, rule-based application of knowledge to the control of food safety and quality.

Put simply, HACCP asks the questions:

- What can go wrong?
- What can I do to prevent things from going wrong?
- What can I do when things do go wrong?

Instead of relying on retrospective microbiological and chemical analyses that are both slow and expensive, HACCP is based on carefully defined control measures such as temperature and time. These controls are easy, quick and cheap to implement and remedial action can be taken before problems occur.

The HACCP approach to assuring food safety is now a proven and internationally recognized system that has been adopted widely across the globe. Some of the good reasons for having a HACCP system in place and the adverse consequences of not having one are listed in Table 9.1. In many countries, food businesses are required to demonstrate a functioning HACCP scheme by law (see Chapter 10).

Table 9.1 Reasons for having a Hazard Analysis and Critical Control Point (HACCP) system

Good reasons for having a HACCP system	Possible adverse consequences of not having a functioning HACCP system
The risks of poisoning customers are reduced	More likely to produce unsafe foods and poison customers
It is an internationally recognized food-safety system that has been shown to work when implemented properly	Reduced confidence in management from Environmental Health Officers (food hygiene inspectors), triggering more frequent inspections
It is preventative. Action is taken before serious problems occur	Risk of business failure due to recalls, complaints, civil action by customers and bad publicity
Food safety is integrated at the product or recipe development stage	More food spoilage and hence wastage
By involving all staff in checking and monitoring the controls, a food-safety culture is generated	Staff fail to recognize that food safety is a shared responsibility leading to complacency and carelessness
Useful for demonstrating due diligence if prosecuted in a court of law	Unlikely to succeed with a due diligence defence in a court of law
It is necessary to comply with the law	More likely to break food-safety laws

HACCP systems are characterized by three key terms: hazard, severity and risk.

A **hazard** is a source of danger. In this book we are focusing on microbiological hazards but hazards can also be physical or chemical. For example, raw ingredients may contain fragments of bone, stones, pips, pieces of metal, plastic or even glass. Organic debris might include animal droppings, feathers, insect wings or whole bodies of pests such as rats and mice. Flakes of paint, nails, wood and glass can chip off walls and equipment into food. As we've seen in Chapter 8, humans and their behaviour can also represent a hazard. Physical hazards associated with humans may include wound dressings, cigarette butts and jewellery. Some foods may be allergenic by their very nature, for example peanuts, milk, fish, wheat and eggs all contain proteins that can provoke an allergic reaction in some people. Segregation of these foods can be difficult and so allergen control is often dependent on clear labelling and good communication with the customer.

A hazard has the potential to cause ill health or even death. A hazard can occur during primary production on the farm, manufacturing, distribution, catering, retailing or consumer use. A hazard is assessed in terms of severity and risk.

Severity is the level of danger presented by the hazard. For example, an incorrectly processed can of pork represents a very severe hazard because botulism is a serious food-poisoning illness that can kill people. Raw oysters are a less severe hazard because infections with norovirus or *Vibrio parahaemolyticus* are relatively mild diseases.

Risk is an estimate of the likely occurrence of a hazard. Since risk is difficult to quantify, foods are often ranked as high risk, medium risk or low risk. For example, canned foods are low risk because the 'botulinum cook' used in most modern canning factories ensures that botulism is now relatively rare. However, oysters are a high-risk food because they are often consumed without cooking, which would otherwise eliminate many food pathogens that may be present.

To sum up the above examples, commercially canned pork is a severe hazard but is a low-risk food. On the other hand, oysters represent a less severe hazard but are a high-risk food. For more information on botulism, norovirus and *Vibrio* infections, see Chapter 7.

Before a new HACCP system is introduced in any food business, certain conditions have to be met. These conditions are known as Prerequisite Programmes and include procedures for hygienic building design, equipment maintenance and calibration, work flow patterns, receiving and storage of goods, staff training, cleaning and disinfection, pest control, waste management and product recall. These Prerequisite Programmes need to be documented and updated at least annually. Once these are in place, a HACCP system can be developed.

The requirements of a HACCP plan need not be daunting. A HACCP plan can be broken down into two stages each consisting of a series of steps as follows:

Stage 1 (five steps)

1 *Assemble a HACCP team.* The success of every HACCP plan depends on a team effort. Without this, the plan will not work. HACCP team members may require specific training in addition to their standard food-hygiene training. The team should include managers as well as non-technical staff.

2 *Describe the food product.* What is the product and its composition? What are the likely uses of the product by the end user or consumer? What are the potential misuses of the product after it leaves the control of the producer?

3 *Identify the intended use.* Likely customers could be from the general population in which one in six might be more vulnerable to infection. Vulnerable groups include young children, the elderly, pregnant women or people on immuno-suppressing drugs. In an institution such as a care home for the elderly, 100 per cent of the customers are in a vulnerable group.

4 *Construct a flow diagram.* All steps in a food-processing operation need to be included, from the purchase of raw materials through to dispatch or service and consumption by the customer. The steps need to describe details such as

Box 9.1 Flow diagram for vichyssoise soup

Amount: 50 L

Ingredients (specify weight and/or volume of each):

- butter;
- onions;
- potatoes;
- vegetable stock;
- milk;
- salt and pepper;
- parsley (as garnish).

Shelf life: serve on day of preparation and up to 2 days thereafter.

Likely use: serve hot or cold.

Intended use: restaurant diners drawn from general population.

Method of preparation

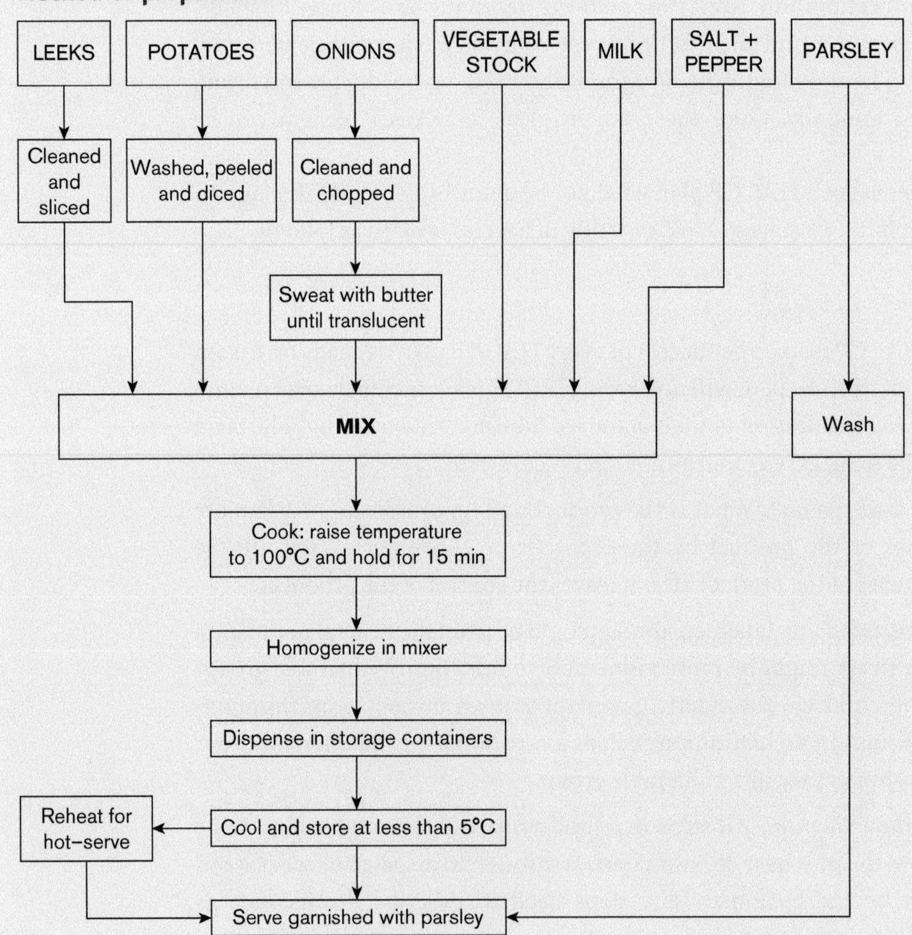

weights, volumes, exact temperatures and times of cooking, cooling and storage. The first draft is usually prepared on paper in an office but it then needs to be verified on the premises where the food is prepared. An example of a first draft of a flow chart for vichyssoise (leek and potato) soup served in a medium-sized restaurant is shown in Box 9.1.

5 *Confirm the flow diagram.* All members of the HACCP team take the flow chart to the food preparation premises during normal operating times and check that the steps are accurately described. The flow diagram is corrected on site. This is essential as flow diagrams must reflect what actually happens, not what the manager thinks is happening. Flow diagrams need to be reviewed regularly and especially when individual steps are omitted or substituted with other steps.

Once a flow diagram has been verified, the second stage of HACCP analysis can be done as follows.

Stage 2 (seven steps)

1. *Identify the hazards and the measures needed to control the hazards.*
2. *Determine the Critical Control Points (CCPs)* in the process. There may be many Control Points in a process but only some of them will be Critical or essential to prevent a food-safety hazard or reduce it to an acceptable level.
3. *Establish the critical limits* for each CCP
4. *Establish a system for monitoring* each CCP
5. *Establish the corrective action* needed if a CCP is not under control
6. *Establish procedures for verification* to confirm that the HACCP system is working
7. *Establish procedures for generating documentation.* Written records of all measures taken in Steps 1–6 must be kept.

An example of a HACCP chart for the vichyssoise soup is shown in Table 9.2.

As shown in Table 9.2, food preparation begins with the purchase of the ingredients. Food is traded in a global market and ingredients are sourced from all over the world. When sourcing ingredients, traceability is important. If the source of a food ingredient is not known, it is not possible to know whether it has been produced to the highest standards.

It is often said that a chef's dishes and reputation are only as secure as the standards of the weakest supplier. Similarly, the health of the customers eating in restaurants, institutions or from supermarkets depends on the safety standards of the weakest supplier of those establishments. Many large supermarket chains protect their brands and reputations by specifying strict food-safety requirements in their purchasing contracts (more on this in Chapter 10). When purchasing food

Table 9.2 Example of a Hazard Analysis and Critical Control Point (HACCP) chart for vichyssoise soup (this table is to be read in conjunction with Box 9.1)

Processing step	Hazard/s	Controls	Is it a Critical Control Point?	Critical limits	Monitoring	Corrective action	Who is responsible?
Purchase	Contamination by pathogenic and spoilage microbes	Use a reputable or approved supplier	No	Certificates of quality	Check certificates, visit supplier if possible	Change the supplier	Manager
Transport and delivery	Microbes multiply	Refrigerated vehicles for milk and butter, maximum 8°C; move from vehicles to chill storage within 15 minutes of delivery	No	8°C on delivery; target temperature 5°C	On delivery check: temperatures, date marks, excessive dirt on vegetables	Reject all goods out of date or dirty/damaged; reject all chilled foods if temperature exceeds 8°C	Person taking deliveries
Storage	Microbes continue to multiply; cross-contamination by raw animal products (e.g. meat)	Refrigerate milk and butter at 5°C; separate from raw meats; rotate stock	No	Chilled foods at 8°C; target 5°C	Check and record temperatures twice per day; check date marks	Discard foods past their date marks or with signs of spoilage	Food handler
Preparation	Microbes continue to grow; new microbes added by food handlers	Maintain good personal hygiene and cleaning protocols	No	Maximum time for chilled foods at ambient temperatures: 30 minutes	Auditing at regular intervals; visual checks of cleaning schedules	Discard foods with signs of spoilage or chilled foods at 8°C or more for 4 hours	Food handler/supervisor

Cooking	Survival of some microbes, especially spores	Heat to 95–100°C and cook for 15 minutes	Yes	95°C (target 75°C) for 15 minutes	Check temperature using a thermometer and timer	Continue heating until food reaches 75°C throughout	Food handler
Cooling	Microbes that survive the cooking multiply	Begin within 30 minutes of cooking completion; use blast chiller to move through danger zone (5–63°C) quickly	Yes	No more than 2 hours (target 90 minutes) to reach 10°C or less	Check temperature using a thermometer and timer	Discard if at 10°C for 2 hours or more	Food handler/ supervisor
Chill storage	Cold-tolerant microbes multiply; others survive	Refrigerate below 5°C; separate cooked foods from raw meats	Yes	Maximum 4 hours at 8°C; target 5°C	Check and record temperature twice per day	Discard if at more than 8°C for 4 hours or more	Food handler/ supervisor
Prepare for serving cold	Microbes multiply; contamination by food handlers	No more than 20 minutes at room temperature	Yes	30 minutes at room temperature	Audit at regular intervals	Discard if at more than 8°C for 2 hours	Supervisor
Reheat	Microbes survive	Reheat to 75°C or more for 2 minutes with stirring	Yes	75°C	Check temperature using a thermometer	Continue heating until temperature reaches 75°C	Food handler
Prepare for serving hot	Microbes multiply	Serve immediately for consumption within 20 minutes or hot-hold at 63°C	Yes	63°C for maximum 2 hours	Audit at regular intervals	Discard after 2 hours at 63°C	Food handler/ supervisor

ingredients, ask yourself: Do you know who your suppliers are and can you trust them?

The acceptability of a supplier can be assessed by personal visits or employment of Hygiene Officers to inspect the premises. If this is not practical, copies of the supplier's HACCP plans or other evidence of good hygienic practice as well as quality certificates can be requested.

Cheaper ingredients can mean inferior ingredients. A purchasing policy that relies on price alone is a recipe for disaster. A food business that adopts a purchasing policy based entirely on costs may be deemed negligent in the event of a food-poisoning outbreak occurring as a result of contaminated food.

There are many generic control measures that can be used in a food-preparation environment but how does one decide which Control Points are critically important for a HACCP plan? In the vichyssoise example given in Table 9.2, multiplication of food-poisoning microbes could occur during any of the early steps including distribution, storage and preparation of the ingredients. Good storage of vegetables in a dry store will avoid premature spoilage as will chill storage of ingredients such as butter and milk. Good hygienic practices during preparation of the vegetables are also desirable. However, it is the cooking step that will destroy most food pathogens that may be present in the soup mixture. Therefore, the cooking step is a **Critical Control Point** in the HACCP plan. Since the soup will be eaten cold by some customers (both hot and cold options are on offer), all subsequent steps including rapid cooling, good chill storage of the cooked soup and avoidance of cross-contamination are also Critical Control Points.

The cooking step is often an obvious Critical Control Point in many HACCP plans. Both the temperature and the holding time at a specified temperature can be set, monitored and corrected. However, time/temperature combinations are not the only Control Points available to the food professional. Acidity (pH), water activity and salt content are examples of some of the other control options available. For more on control, go back to Chapter 8!

Before the advent of digital temperature probes for foods, the recommendation 'cook meat until juices run clear' was often used. This was a qualitative measure based on the fact that blood coagulates (solidifies) at 74°C. Modern food-processing operations no longer rely on such subjective assessment of temperature. It is now an expectation that all food businesses will have in place a means of monitoring temperature accurately. Many inexpensive temperature measuring devices are now available for use in food-preparation areas and include those suitable for use in cooked meats. Recommended temperatures for cooking meat in the UK and the US are shown in Box 8.2.

As we've seen in Chapters 7 and 8, heating food at 75°C or above is an excellent way of killing off vegetative bacterial cells but has no effect on heat-resistant spores (see also Fig. 8.5). Since cooking creates an anaerobic atmosphere, cooling time must be minimized to prevent spores of *Clostridium* and *Bacillus* from germinating and producing toxins. Once a food is fully cooked, the following rules apply:

- Hot-served foods must be kept above 63°C but only for a period of no more than 2 hours.
- Cold-served foods must be cooled to 5°C within 90 minutes of cooking completion.

These simple rules are helpful when setting the critical limits (Step 3 above) for each Control Point in a HACCP plan. The limits separate the acceptable from the unacceptable. Critical limits are often expressed as combinations of temperature and time. For example, if the critical limit for storing a chilled food is 8°C for 4 hours and the temperature reaches 9°C, then the food becomes unacceptable. The food also becomes unacceptable if kept at 8°C for longer than 4 hours. Once a food is deemed unacceptable, it must be thrown away. In practice, refrigeration targets are set below the critical limits so that potential breaches of the critical limits can be detected early and corrected before the food becomes unfit to eat. For example, a target of 5°C and a critical limit of 8°C for 4 hours could be set for a refrigerator. If the temperature creeps up to 6°C or 7°C during a busy service period or following delivery of new batches of food, corrective action can be taken by adjusting the thermostat. In this way, the processing step is brought back under control and food wastage is avoided. The difference between a target and a critical limit is often referred to as tolerance.

Automatic data loggers fitted with alarms are preferable to manual monitoring of temperatures in refrigerators and freezers but these are generally available only in the larger and more modern food-processing establishments.

HACCP plans need to be reviewed regularly and especially when changes are made to the recipe or the individual steps in the process. New scientific information about foodborne illness and revised public health guidelines can also trigger reviews of HACCP systems.

The paperwork needed to support HACCP systems is seen by some as onerous and time consuming, particularly for small food businesses. The amount of documentation generated should be appropriate for the size and type of the business. A small newsagent selling pre-packed chocolate bars does not require the same approach as a large food manufacturer producing several thousand chicken and leek pies per day.

HACCP documentation should include the charts generated by Stages 1 and 2 above, monitoring records, lists of approved suppliers and records of staff training, sickness, equipment calibration and maintenance, and customer complaints. Without efficient record-keeping it is impossible for food inspectors (Environmental Health Officers) to audit food-preparation practices. Many auditors follow the principle of 'If it isn't written down, it doesn't exist'. It's no good claiming that fridge temperatures get checked twice per day if no record exists to prove that this happens. Good record-keeping can also help to protect the business in the event of a food-poisoning outbreak by demonstrating that all possible care has been taken to assure food-safety practices. This is known as a **due diligence** defence in a court of law.

While it is instructive to see an example of a HACCP plan, every food operation is different and consequently requires a customized plan. In drawing up their HACCP plans, food-business operators often need help with differentiating between Control Points and Critical Control Points. Such help is available internationally from the Codex Alimentarius Commission and from national organizations. In the UK, the Food Standards Agency has developed resources and tools available free-of-charge to help food businesses to implement a HACCP-based approach. For a list of helpful websites, see Weblinks section below:

Chapter 9 Exercise

Choose a food operation used in your workplace or select a recipe that involves a cooking step and prepare a HACCP plan for it. Start by drawing a flow diagram similar to the one shown in Box 9.1. Follow the steps in Stage 1 and prepare a HACCP chart like the example shown in Table 9.2 using Steps 1 through 6 in Stage 2. Discuss with your supervisor at work and/or students in class.

Further reading

Taylor, E and Taylor, JZ (2004). Safer Food, Better Business: A new HACCP methodology for catering. *Food Science and Technology* **18 (3)**, 22–5.

Taylor, JZ, Assan, N, Green, R, McCann, J and Rodriguez, J (2008). Menu-safe: A new method of HACCP for the hospitality industry: Embracing new cuisines and developing sector relevance. *International Journal of Contemporary Hospitality Management* **20 (5)**, 561–78.

Wallace, C (2009). Intermediate HACCP, 3rd edn. Highfield Publications, UK (may be purchased from: **http://www. highfield. co. uk**).

Weblinks

Safer Food, Better Business is a jargon-free, simplified hygiene pack intended for small catering businesses such as restaurants, cafés and takeaways. The four C's (Cross-contamination, Cleaning, Chilling and Cooking) and their

management are explained and illustrated with colour photographs of foods and correct hygiene procedures. Personal hygiene, pest control and equipment maintenance are also included as are several generic templates for food-safety management and record-keeping. The pack has been adapted for Chinese, Indian, Pakistani, Bangladeshi and Sri Lankan cuisines and is available in 16 languages. Supplements are available for residential care homes and childminders. The pack can be viewed online and downloaded from:
http://www. food. gov. uk/foodindustry/regulation/hygleg/hyglegresources/sfbb/
and
http://www. sfbbtraining. co. uk/

An 8-minute video demonstrating the importance of good food hygiene, *Bacteria Bites Business*, is available on:
http://www. flyonthewall. com/FlyBroadcast/FSA/BacteriaBiteBusiness/

The *Safe Catering* guide, developed by Northern Ireland's Food Standards Agency in collaboration with the food industry and local authorities is more comprehensive than *Safer Food Better Business* and intended for a wider range of food businesses. Issue 4 was updated in 2007 and is available from:
http://www. food. gov. uk/northernireland/safetyhygieneni/safecateringni/

The Scottish Food Standards Agency has produced a helpful pack for the catering trade known as *CookSafe*. It comes in English as well as Chinese, Bengali, Punjabi and Urdu. Additional support for the hard-copy manual is available electronically as *e-CookSafe*. Similarly, *RetailSafe* was designed for retailers handling unwrapped high-risk foods such as those sold from fresh meat and fish counters and in-store delicatessens. These resources are available from:
http://www. food. gov. uk/foodindustry/regulation/hygleg/hyglegresources/cookretailscotland/cooksafe/
and
http://www. food. gov. uk/foodindustry/regulation/hygleg/hyglegresources/cookretailscotland/retailsafe/

The WHO and the Industry Council for Development have published a comprehensive 600-page training manual on HACCP intended to support a 4-day training course for food-industry personnel and food inspectors. The manual includes lecture slides, flow diagrams and case studies on fried chicken, a fresh-cream gateau and dried milk. It is available online, in hard copy or on CD-ROM at:
http://www. who. int/foodsafety/publications/fs_management/haccp_teachers/en/#

The US Department of Agriculture (Food Safety Inspection Service) has produced a guidebook for the preparation of HACCP plans and several models for specific foods in English and Spanish. These are available from:
http://www. fsis. usda. gov/Science/Generic_HACCP_Models/index. asp

The Canadian Food Inspection Service also provides a comprehensive manual on HACCP and a generic model for poultry slaughter. These are available from:
http://www. inspection. gc. ca/english/fssa/polstrat/haccp/manue/tablee. shtml
and
http://www. inspection. gc. ca/english/fssa/polstrat/haccp/haccpe. shtml

For fish and seafood guides and HACCP plans, the Seafood Network Information Center hosted by the University of California Davis is useful:
http://seafood. ucdavis. edu/seafoodhaccp. html
and
http://seafood. ucdavis. edu/haccp/compendium/compend. htm

Legislation and maintaining standards

The law

In the UK, the Food Safety Act 1990 and its amendments (see Box 10.1) provide the framework for all food legislation. The main aim of this framework is to protect human health and consumers in relation to food.

Put simply, the law makes it illegal to sell food that is 'injurious to health or unfit for human consumption'. Food shall not be placed on the market if it is unsafe.

Furthermore, the presentation of the food (labelling, advertising, display) must not mislead consumers. All foods entering and leaving a food business must be traceable. In other words, food-business operators are required to keep records of foods, food ingredients and food-producing animals supplied to their businesses

Box 10.1 Main food-safety laws in the UK

The Food Safety Act 1990

The General Food Law Regulation (EC) 178/2002

The General Food Regulations 2004
(Amendment of the Food Safety Act 1990 to bring it in line with European Regulation 178/2002)

The Food Standards Agency (FSA) in the UK has developed two jargon-free guides for businesses regarding food-safety law. These are downloadable from:

http://food. gov. uk/multimedia/pdfs/fsactguide. pdf
The Food Safety Act 1990 – A Guide for Food Businesses, 2009.

http://food. gov. uk/multimedia/pdfs/fsa1782002guidance. pdf
Guidance notes for food-business operators on food safety, traceability, withdrawals and recall. A guide to compliance with articles 14, 16, 18 and 19 of General Food Law Regulation (EC) 178/2002, 2007.

and of food products dispatched to other businesses. These records must be available for inspection by authorities on demand. Foods that are not in compliance with food-safety requirements must be withdrawn from sale or recalled if they have already reached the consumer.

All food-business premises must be registered with their local authority. Anyone starting a new food business must register 28 days before opening.

Breaking any of the food laws is an offence and can be prosecuted. The level of penalties is decided by the courts depending on the circumstances of each case but the Act allows for unlimited fines and imprisonment of up to 2 years.

In addition to the general principles of food law laid out in the Food Safety Act 1990, there are numerous specific regulations concerning hygiene, milk and milk products, meat and meat products, fish and fish products, bread and flour, cocoa and chocolate, coffee, fruit juices, jam, honey, bottled water, addition of vitamins, animal feed, novel foods, food additives, packaging materials, labelling, etc. The list is seemingly endless. The most important of these for all food businesses is European *Regulation (EC) 852/2004* on the hygiene of foodstuffs (see weblink at end of chapter). The food-hygiene regulation was an attempt to harmonize a multitude (17 to be exact) of separate European Union measures concerning food hygiene. Additional regulations 853/2004 for food businesses dealing with foods of animal origin and 854/2004 relating to official controls of animal products supplement the main regulation.

In the UK, Regulation (EC) 852/2004 is implemented as The Food Hygiene (England) Regulation 2006 with equivalent country-specific regulations operating in Scotland, Wales and Northern Ireland. The European Union regulation replaced two old UK regulations, namely the 1995 Food Safety (General Food Hygiene) Regulation and the Food Safety (Temperature Control) Regulation 2005. The food-hygiene regulation came into force in the UK in January 2006. All 27 Member States of the European Union have also implemented the regulation in each country.

The regulation sets out basic hygiene requirements for all food businesses including primary producers (farmers and growers). Crucially, Article 5 of the regulation states that all food businesses must implement and maintain food-safety management procedures based on Hazard Analysis Critical Control Point (HACCP) principles and so it is sometimes referred to as the HACCP law. The regulation stipulates the very stringent HACCP requirements developed by Codex Alimentarius although some flexibility is acceptable for very small low-risk businesses.

The Codex Alimentarius Commission is an international body formed in the 1960s to implement the joint Food and Agriculture Organization (FAO) and World Health Organization (WHO) Food Standards Programme. The main objective of the programme is to protect the health of consumers and to set internationally agreed standards for foods known as Codex Standards (see weblink at end of chapter). In 2011 there were 183 Member States in the Codex Commission.

In practice, it is expected that HACCP procedures are proportionate to the size and nature of the business. Once a HACCP system is in place, it must be adhered to permanently, reviewed regularly and documented so that records can be checked by enforcement officers. For further details on HACCP, see Chapter 9.

The areas covered by the regulation are summarized in Table 10.1 and the original document can be obtained from the weblink at the end of the chapter. A jargon-free guide for restaurants, cafés and other catering businesses as well as shops selling food is available from the UK Food Standards Agency (FSA) on:

http://www. food. gov. uk/multimedia/pdfs/publication/hygieneguidebooklet. pdf *Food hygiene: A guide for businesses. Information on regulations and good practice*. Revised June 2011.

Good temperature control features prominently in the European hygiene regulation but exact temperatures for cooking, chilling and freezing are not specified. Consequently, specific requirements regarding temperatures can vary from country to country and must be checked before adopting in a local business. In the UK, the law says that:

- *Cold food must be kept at 8°C or below.* During food preparation at ambient temperatures, chilled foods may be allowed to exceed 8°C for up to 4 hours. However, this must not be done more than once. After this period, the food must go back in the fridge or be discarded. In practice, many businesses aim to keep their chilled foods at 5°C in order to allow a margin for corrective action and avoid having to discard a lot of food. For further details on how this is done within a HACCP plan, see Chapter 9. It is good practice to store chilled foods at 5°C.
- *Hot food must be kept at 63°C or above.* Hot food may be kept on a hot-serve counter or carvery at this temperature for up to 2 hours. This should only be done once. After this period, any remaining food should be discarded or reheated as set out below and put back into hot holding.
- When reheating food, it must be piping hot (steaming) all the way through (or must reach 82°C in Scotland).

The law does not specify cooking times and temperatures but the FSA in the UK recommends the following core temperatures and minimum times:

- 60°C for 45 minutes;
- 65°C for 10 minutes;
- 70°C for 2 minutes;
- 75°C for 30 seconds;
- 80°C for 6 seconds.

Table 10.1 Legal requirements of Regulation EC852/2004 on the hygiene of foodstuffs

Chapter	Title	Requirements
1	The premises (all rooms and buildings used for the food business)	Must be clean and in good repair Layout, design and site must promote hygienic food handling by: • minimizing opportunities for contamination from air, pests, cleaning chemicals, etc. • allowing for easy cleaning, disinfection and maintenance • providing enough working space, lighting, ventilation and drainage • providing good temperature control where appropriate with good monitoring and recording Staff facilities must include: • toilets not opening directly into food handling areas • dedicated hand wash basins with hot and cold water, soap and drying facilities • changing room/area
2	Food-preparation rooms	Layout and design must promote good hygienic practices and protect against contamination between and during tasks There are requirements for: • floors, walls, ceilings, windows, doors and all surfaces including food-contact surfaces • facilities for washing food • facilities for cleaning, disinfecting and storing utensils and equipment
3	Mobile and temporary premises and private dwellings where food is prepared for sale	Must include facilities for: maintaining personal hygiene (toilets, hand washing, changing), supplying hot and cold potable (drinking-quality) water, cleaning and disinfection, waste disposal, appropriate food-contact surfaces, temperature control and avoidance of cross-contamination
4	Transport	Food containers and vehicles must prevent contamination by separating products effectively, cleaning between loads and temperature control
5	Equipment	Food-processing equipment must be made of appropriate materials, installed correctly and kept in good repair. Equipment must be cleaned and disinfected when appropriate. Control devices such as temperature sensors must be fitted

Fitness to work is another important aspect of the European food-hygiene regulation. Food handlers (except those working in primary production) suffering from diarrhoea or wound and skin infections should not be permitted to work. The food handlers themselves have a responsibility to tell their managers when they are ill and the managers have a duty to exclude infected people from work. To help businesses meet their legal obligations, the FSA has produced guidelines on determining food handlers' fitness to work. A weblink to these guidelines is provided at the end of this chapter. In brief, the FSA recommends that food handlers should report symptoms such as diarrhoea, vomiting, nausea, stomach

Chapter	Title	Requirements
6	Food waste	Standards for removal, storage and disposal of food waste are laid out including the design of waste containers and waste storage areas
7	Water supply	Potable (drinking-quality) water must be used for all food processing, ice and steam for heating foods. Conditions when non-potable water may be used are specified
8	Personal hygiene	Food handlers must: • practice a high level of personal cleanliness • wear suitable clean or protective clothing • not handle food if they have infected wounds, skin infections or diarrhoea • inform their manager of illness or symptoms
9	Food	Control systems must be in place for: • receiving and storing raw materials and ingredients • protecting food from contamination during preparation and distribution • pest control • temperature control • thawing of frozen products • separation of hazardous chemicals from food
10	Wrapping and packaging	Materials must not be a source of contamination and must be stored appropriately. Re-usable containers must be easy to clean and disinfect if necessary
11	Heating	Must be controlled to ensure that all parts of the food have received the correct temperature treatment and that cross-contamination is avoided post-treatment. Processes must be monitored and validated
12	Training	Staff must be supervised and instructed or trained in food hygiene at a level appropriate to their job responsibilities. Person responsible for food-safety management based on HACCP must have received adequate training

HACCP, Hazard Analysis Critical Control Point.

ache, fever, jaundice and skin infections to their managers as soon as they occur. Managers then need to exclude the infected handler from working with or around open food. In larger businesses, this might involve moving the handler to a different role (e.g. to work in reception in a hotel) for a few days but in small businesses complete absence from work may be necessary. Absence due to sickness should not be penalized by withdrawing pay as this may encourage employees to hide their symptoms. The FSA recommends that staff with diarrhoea or vomiting should not return to work involving food handling until they have had no symptoms for 48 hours.

According to the regulation, it is a legal requirement for food handlers to receive hygiene training appropriate for the work that they do. However, there is no legal requirement for staff to attend a formal or accredited training course or have formal qualifications. The necessary skills can be obtained through on-the-job training, work experience or self-study. In practice, it can be more difficult to prove that staff have adequate skills in food hygiene unless they have received formal training and a certificate. The corollary is, of course, also true in that paper qualifications are no guarantee that all staff practice good hygiene at a satisfactory level. Nevertheless, many businesses now require all staff to attend basic training and encourage some to gain more advanced qualifications. For some of the training courses and qualifications available, see Table 8.7.

Meeting the requirement for trained staff can represent a challenge for food businesses where there is a high turnover of employees. Untrained staff can be a liability. In addition, training alone is often not sufficient to change behaviour. Good hygienic practices must become part of the culture of any food establishment to achieve real gains in food safety. In other words, the law is not enough to ensure a safe food supply.

The main defence that a food business can use in a court of law is that of **due diligence**. To use this defence, the business owner, company or food trader must prove that they have taken all reasonable care to avoid committing an offence. The courts decide what 'reasonable care' is in each case. The defence of due diligence can be used under the general food-law framework as well as under the specific food-hygiene regulations. For an example of what can happen when food laws are broken, see Box 10.2. Other examples are given in pp. 5, 43, 81.

Box 10.2 Fish-shop owner jailed

The owner of a fish and chip takeaway shop was jailed for 8 months in 2011 for causing a food-poisoning outbreak that made nine people ill. Four people were taken to hospital with *E. coli* 0157:H7 poisoning and one required intensive care.

The fish-shop owner had previously been warned about poor hygiene in his establishment but had chosen to ignore the warnings and the advice of the Environmental Health Practitioner (food inspector). The owner admitted that he had failed to separate raw from cooked foods adequately and had neglected to implement a Hazard Analysis Critical Control Point (HACCP) plan, despite receiving training. Furthermore, foods were not properly protected from insects and an electrical fly killer was not working. The hand wash basin in the staff toilet was not available for its intended use because it was used as a place for storing clothes.

In addition to the jail sentence, the owner was banned from running a food business ever again.

Enforcement of the law

In the UK, FSA is responsible for food policy, legislation and guidance but enforcement is delegated to local government authorities. The 434 local authorities in the UK are responsible for inspecting over half a million food establishments, of which nearly 90 per cent employ 10 or fewer people. The preponderance of small businesses in the food sector is similar in other European countries. Consequently, the European Commission allows some flexibility and proportionality for small businesses implementing the food-hygiene regulation and HACCP. In the UK, the FSA has collaborated with the local authorities and industry to produce helpful guides such as the Safer Food Better Business pack (see Chapter 9 for weblink) in an effort to assist small businesses to comply with the law.

Food law is enforced by Environmental Health Practitioners (EHPs) or Officers (EHOs) and Trading Standards Officers (TSOs) who are employed by local authorities. EHPs are principally responsible for hygiene and microbiological and chemical contamination of foods. TSOs are responsible for labelling and legal use of ingredients. Both EHPs and TSOs disseminate information about national food-safety alerts to local businesses and consumers.

Local authorities undertake routine inspections of food businesses on a regular basis. In addition, an inspection may be triggered by a customer complaint. An EHP has the right to enter the business at any reasonable time of day and usually arrives unannounced.

During an inspection, an EHP first makes a thorough visual assessment of the premises and equipment. This includes attention to:

- design of the premises and layout;
- workflow patterns;
- lighting and ventilation;
- pest-proofing;
- staff toilets and washrooms: hand-washing facilities, including hot and cold water, soap, drying facilities, hand-hygiene reminders;
- dishwashing facilities, temperature of hot water/dishwasher cycle;
- waste storage, indoors and out;
- temperature control during cooking;
- temperature control of refrigerators and freezers;
- measures to minimize cross-contamination from raw to ready-to-eat or cooked foods;
- staff training and commitment to food-safety practices.

Some of the potential problems that an EHP may look out for include:

- inadequate cooking, that is, failure to reach adequate temperatures when cooking or re-heating high-risk foods such as meat (see Box 8.2);
- cooling foods too slowly after cooking;
- failing to maintain the chill chain, e.g. faulty refrigerators/thermostats, chill foods kept at ambient temperatures for too long;
- long delays between preparation and consumption, especially when catering for large functions such as weddings;
- opportunities for cross-contamination through insufficient separation of raw and cooked foods during storage, and via hands, utensils, chopping boards and sinks;
- potential contamination of foods by infected handlers – effective exclusion or fitness to work policy.

An EHP makes observations and has an in-depth discussion with the staff to determine what actually happens during food preparation. Particular attention is paid to training and supervision to determine if managers and staff are capable of running a business safely. The nature and volume of the business are taken into account as is the potential vulnerability of the customer group. The EHP also examines the documentation, including HACCP charts (see Chapter 9) kept by the food business.

Most EHPs do not just inspect food businesses but also provide information and advice on improving existing standards of hygiene. The EHP may also offer free resource packs and alert businesses to health education programmes and lectures organized locally. These actions are intended to be helpful and are taken before resorting to the punitive arm of the law.

EHPs are authorized to take photographs and samples of food or surface swabs for analysis, and copy or seize written records. If the food business is not complying with the law, the EHP can issue an **Improvement Notice** or written warning specifying what action needs to be taken within a specified time period. Alternatively, if the breaches of food-safety law are so serious that they represent an imminent danger to the public, the EHP can issue a **Prohibition Notice** that effectively closes down the business until remedial action has been taken. In addition, the EHP may initiate prosecution in a court of law that may lead to an unlimited fine, imprisonment up to 2 years and a permanent ban from running a food business ever again.

Scores on the Doors schemes: encouraging self-regulation

Hygiene rating schemes are increasingly being used around the world to encourage food businesses to improve their practices without resorting to the strong arm of the law. Publication of hygiene ratings allows consumers to make informed choices about where to dine or purchase their food. Consumer choice, the power of the customer and peer (or competitor) pressure provide a strong incentive for businesses to drive up hygiene standards.

In the UK, several pilot schemes using different scoring scales were tested in the mid-2000s. In December 2008, the FSA announced a national scheme based on 5 stars for England, Wales and Northern Ireland (see Boxes 10.3 and 10.4). Scotland retains a rating scheme based on 'pass/improvement required'. Known as the 'Scores on the Doors' scheme, the national programme captured more than 150 000 restaurants, pubs, shops, cafés, hotels, supermarkets, clubs and takeaways by mid-2011. As more local authorities join the scheme, it is hoped that the majority of food businesses will be included before the review planned by the FSA for 2012.

Following a food-hygiene inspection by the local Environmental Health Practitioner, each business is awarded a star rating. The rating is based on three elements: hygiene and safety; the structure of the premises; and confidence in management. The business is given a certificate and a window sticker showing the rating.

Display of the ratings is not compulsory but all ratings are published on the Internet on a dedicated website (http://www. scoresonthedoors. org. uk) that can also be accessed via mobile devices. Clearly, food businesses with high ratings are likely to display their scores prominently, while those with low ratings may choose not to do so. Nevertheless, the absence of a hygiene score display allows consumers to draw their own conclusions. Furthermore, many restaurant critics now include the hygiene star rating in their reviews. In the meantime, many local authorities and consumer organizations are lobbying the FSA for a mandatory requirement to display scores.

Box 10.3 Scores on the Doors: UK food-hygiene rating

*****	Excellent. Very high standards of food-safety management. Fully compliant with food-safety legislation.
****	Very good. Good food-safety management. High standard of compliance with food-safety legislation.
***	Good. Good level of legal compliance. Some more effort might be required.
**	Broadly compliant. Broadly compliant with food-safety legislation. More effort required to meet all legal requirements.
*	Poor. Poor level of compliance with food-safety legislation. Much more effort required.
No stars	Very poor. A general failure to comply with legal requirements. Little or no appreciation of food safety. Major effort required.

Box 10.4 Restaurant awarded zero stars

A local restaurant has received no stars following a food-hygiene inspection by the local council's food-safety team. The owner of the restaurant was fined £6000 and ordered to pay £380 in court costs after pleading guilty to four food-hygiene offences.

Food-hygiene inspectors found thick black grease on the floor, staff dressed in dirty overalls, uncovered food lying around and dirty work surfaces.

As part of the Scores on the Doors scheme, the hygiene rating was published on the Internet. Several stories about the restaurant's hygiene failures were also reported in the local press.

Many countries operate hygiene rating schemes. For example, in Denmark, food inspectors award one of four scores illustrated by a 'smiley face'. A very happy smiley indicates that the food inspector had no remarks; a moderately happy smiley indicates that certain rules must be obeyed; a neutral face indicates that a prohibition order has been issued; and a sour face indicates that the business has been fined, reported to the police or has had its approval withdrawn. The Danish scheme has been in operation since 2001 but in 2008, a new 'elite smiley' score was introduced to reward those businesses receiving happy smileys in four consecutive inspections. Unlike in the UK, displaying the Danish smiley rating is compulsory and full inspection reports are published online (see weblink at end of chapter).

In the USA, many states and cities have their own hygiene rating schemes. For example, New York grades some 24 000 restaurants in the city using a points-based system ranging from 0 to over 28. The points are then translated into grades A, B or C with the most hygienic establishments awarded an A. Grade cards must be posted by the business in a place where they can be seen easily by passers-by (see weblink at end of chapter). Many large cities across the world have their own hygiene scoring schemes in place.

The US Centers for Disease Control and Prevention (CDC) has operated a hygiene inspection scheme for cruise ships since the 1970s. The aim of the Vessel Sanitation Program is to protect both passengers and crew on cruise ships from gastrointestinal illness. Vessels are scored on a points system of 0 to 100. Ships with scores above 86 are classified as satisfactory and placed on the 'green list'. The scores, together with information on best practice and the latest outbreaks on cruise ships are published online (for weblink, see end of chapter).

Food quality and microbiological criteria

What is quality?

The Oxford English dictionary defines quality as a

'degree of excellence, relative nature, or kind, or character'.

Microbiological food quality encompasses microbiological safety, acceptability in terms of shelf life and consistency. These terms are defined as follows:

- *safety*: must *not* contain levels of a pathogen or its toxin likely to cause illness.
- *acceptability/shelf-life*: must *not* contain levels of microorganisms likely to spoil sensory properties of food in an unacceptably short time.
- *consistency*: no large batch-to-batch variations in shelf life and safety.

What is the difference between good-quality and poor-quality foods? Microbiological criteria were developed in an attempt to answer this question. There is a need to distinguish between acceptable and unacceptable food quality. To this end, there are three types of microbiological criteria:

- standards;
- specifications;
- guidelines.

A **standard** is specified by law and enforced by regulatory agencies. For example, milk standards were introduced in the UK in 1982. Farmers were told that the bacterial count in raw milk was too high and that better hygienic practices on the farm would reduce the count. They were then paid less for their milk by the Milk Marketing Board if the count exceeded specified limits. Within 4 months of introducing the new standard, the bacterial counts dropped dramatically across the country. About three quarters of the milk produced in England now has a count of less than 1000 colony forming units per millilitre (cfu/mL).

A **specification** is a criterion applied in commerce. It is a contractual condition of acceptance set by a food processor or retailer on a supplier. For example, a retailer can specify the maximum number of microbial counts per gram (or cfu/g) for frozen peas supplied by a processor.

A **guideline** is an advisory criterion for microbiological acceptability of a food. Professional bodies and government agencies can set and publish guidelines but there is no obligation by law to stick to them. For example, the Chilled Food Association has produced a guide on the 'Shelf life of ready-to-eat food in relation to *L. monocytogenes*' intended for food businesses (see weblink at end of chapter).

A European Regulation EC 2073/2005 on microbiological criteria for foods came into force at the same time as the Hygiene Regulation 852/2004 in January 2006. Regulation EC 2073/2005 requires food businesses to use the criteria specified in the Regulation's extended annex to verify and validate their food-safety management systems based on HACCP principles.

The regulation lays down food-safety criteria for several important pathogens, such as *Salmonella* and *L. monocytogenes*, particularly in ready-to-eat foods. For example, a ready-to-eat food such as a sandwich is deemed satisfactory if *Salmonella* cannot be detected in 25 g of the food at the point of sale. If, however, *Salmonella* is detected, the food is deemed unacceptable or potentially hazardous.

The regulation also lays down process hygiene or quality criteria, measured in a variety of ways. For example, total bacterial counts known as aerobic colony counts per gram (cfu/g) of a food can be used to categorize a food as satisfactory, acceptable or unsatisfactory. In the sandwich example above, a count of less than 10^3 (1000) cfu/g is satisfactory, a count between 10^3 and 10^4 is acceptable and anything over 10^4 is considered unsatisfactory.

Some public health authorities have taken the regulations further and developed more detailed guidelines. For example, in the UK, the Health Protection Agency (HPA) has published guidelines concerning *Campylobacter*, *E. coli* O157:H7, *Salmonella*, *Shigella*, *Vibrio cholerae* and *V. parahaemolyticus*, *Bacillus* (including *B. cereus* and other species), *C. perfringens*, *L. monocytogenes* and *S. aureus*. Advice on the interpretation of results for hygiene indicator organisms, the likely cause and suggested actions is also provided.

As we have seen in previous chapters, food safety is neither guaranteed nor controlled by microbiological testing of the finished food product. A functioning HACCP-based system is key to demonstrating due diligence. However, microbiological testing can be used to validate and monitor processes and Critical Control Points identified during a HACCP plan.

Since microbes are unevenly distributed throughout a food, microbiological testing is subject to a complex statistical sampling design to ensure that the results are representative of the entire batch. Absolute confidence in quality of a batch of food is only possible if all of it is tested, leaving none to eat! Consequently, decisions are a compromise between practicability and estimate of quality.

The aerobic colony count can be used to measure bacterial load on surfaces (see Chapter 3 for more details on swabbing surfaces quantitatively). There are no laws (as yet) specifying bacterial counts for surfaces but some recommendations and guidelines for maximum surface loads exist. For example, in the UK the HPA deems counts of 10 cfu/cm^2 or less from a cleaned ready-to-eat food preparation surface as acceptable, whereas anything higher than this count would be considered unsatisfactory. The US Department of Agriculture (USDA) considers that the count on food-processing equipment should be 5 cfu/cm^2 or less before work begins. Similar microbial surface counts after cleaning have been advocated by the Swedish Food Standards Agency. Some studies have used a threshold count of 2.5 cfu/cm^2 for evaluating cleaning regimes.

In this chapter, we have focused primarily on UK and European food law. Food legislation may be substantially different in other countries although the principles of HACCP are being widely adopted and enshrined in national and international legislation. In the USA, food legislation is undergoing significant change with the enactment of the Food Safety Modernization Act in January 2011. The aim of the Act is to shift the focus of regulation from responding to food-safety problems to preventing them. Major reforms are anticipated over a period of 18 months to 3 years. Weblinks for keeping up to date with US legislation are provided at the end of the chapter.

Further reading

Sprenger, RA (2009). *Hygiene for management: a text for food safety courses.* Highfield, Doncaster, UK.

Weblinks

UK Food Standards Agency (FSA) guidelines, information, publications

2009. *The Food Safety Act 1990 – A guide for food businesses.* Available from: **http://food. gov. uk/multimedia/pdfs/fsactguide. pdf**

For a summary of food law in the UK, visit: **http://food. gov. uk/foodindustry/regulation/foodlaw/**

2007. Guidance notes for food-business operators on food safety, traceability, withdrawals and recall. A guide to compliance with articles 14, 16, 18 and 19 of General Food Law Regulation (EC) 178/2002. **http://food. gov. uk/multimedia/pdfs/fsa1782002guidance. pdf**

European Regulation on Food Hygiene EC852/2004 is available from: **http://www. food. gov. uk/foodindustry/regulation/europeleg/eufoodhygieneleg** and **http://www. food. gov. uk/multimedia/pdfs/hiojregulation. pdf**

For frequently asked questions on the European food-hygiene legislation: **http://www. food. gov. uk/foodindustry/regulation/hygleg/hygleginfo/foodhygknow/**

For background information to the European food-hygiene legislation: **http://www. food. gov. uk/foodindustry/regulation/europeleg/eufoodhygieneleg/**

Food law inspections and your business. 2006 (revised July 2009). Available in English, Gaelic, Bengali, Chinese, Gujarati, Hindi, Punjabi, Thai, Turkish and Urdu: **http://www. food. gov. uk/multimedia/pdfs/publication/foodlawinspec0310. pdf**

Starting up – your first steps to running a catering business. Revised August 2009 and updated March 2010.
Available in English, Gaelic, Bengali, Chinese, Gujarati, Hindi, Punjabi, Thai, Turkish and Urdu:
http://www. food. gov. uk/multimedia/pdfs/publication/startingup0310a. pdf

Food handlers: fitness to work – a practical guide for food business operators. 2009:
http://www. food. gov. uk/multimedia/pdfs/publication/ foodhandlersireland1009.pdf

UK Health Protection Agency (HPA) guidelines, publications

Guidelines for assessing the safety of ready-to-eat foods placed on the market. 2009. This document is intended primarily for Environmental Health Practitioners and other food-safety professionals with a scientific background. The guidelines are available free of charge from:
http://www. hpa. org. uk/web/HPAwebFile/HPAweb_C/1259151921557

Willis, C, Elviss, N, Aird, H, Fenelon, D and McLauchlin, J (2010). An evaluation of hygiene practices in catering premises at large scale events in the UK with a focus on identifying risks for the Olympics 2012 (available from: **http://www. hpa. org. uk/web/HPAwebFile/HPAweb_C/1287144844852**).

Other useful Weblinks

Codex Alimentarius Commission or Joint FAO/WHO Food Standards Programme:
http://www. who. int/foodsafety/codex/en/

For standards and codes of practice developed by Codex and usually published in at least three languages (and sometimes six), visit:
http://www. codexalimentarius. net/web/index_en. jsp

Chilled Food Association. Guidance on microbiological criteria and safety management for food businesses producing chilled ready-to-eat foods is available from:
http://www. chilledfood. org

Guidelines specifically on the 'Shelf life of ready-to-eat food in relation to *L. monocytogenes*' 2010 on:
http://www. chilledfood. org/Resources/Chilled%20Food%20Association/ Public%20Resources/Shelf%20life%20of%20RTE%20foods%20in%20 relation%20to%20Lm%20FINAL%20v1.1.1%2023%203%2010.pdf
Also gives helpful worked examples such as a 'smoked salmon and watercress sandwich' as well as what to do when changing recipes in 'brie with garlic and herbs'.

The USDA web page on sanitation and quality standards includes standards, specifications and guidelines developed by government agencies and industry as well as resources for developing and interpreting microbiological criteria for foods:
http://riley. nal. usda. gov/nal_display/index. php?info_center=1&tax_level=2&tax_subject=606&topic_id=2363

Information on US food legislation is available from:
http://www. fda. gov/food/foodsafety/FSMA/

The Food Code is available from:
http://www. fda. gov/Food/FoodSafety/RetailFoodProtection/FoodCode/default. htm
and the Code of Federal Regulations CFR21 from:
http://www. accessdata. fda. gov/scripts/cdrh/cfdocs/cfcfr/cfrsearch. cfm

Hygiene rating schemes:

UK:
http:www. scoresonthedoors. org. uk

Denmark:
http://www. findsmiley. dk/en-US/Forside. htm

New York City:
http://www. nyc. gov/html/doh/html/rii/index. shtml

Los Angeles:
http://www. publichealth. lacounty. gov/rating/

The CDC Vessel Sanitation Program publishes hygiene inspection scores for cruise ships on:
http://www. cdc. gov/nceh/vsp/

For help with HACCP, see weblinks in Chapter 9.

11

Epilogue: Future perfect?

There is no doubt that modern food production and manufacturing has transformed the way we eat, mainly for the better. Our hunter-gatherer ancestors survived on a frugal diet of berries, nuts, fruits and the occasional morsel of meat after a successful hunting expedition. Their life expectancy was not much more than 30 years.

Right up to the nineteenth century, the daily diet of the majority of people was monotonous and low in protein and many vitamins. Bread, butter, tea, potatoes and kippers provided the daily fare for many workers in Victorian England with occasional treats of roast pork, bacon and eggs. Fresh fruit and vegetables were a rarity for city dwellers. Life expectancy was around 41 years.

In most developed countries today, people enjoy a huge variety of affordable foods, choosing from tens of thousands of different product lines available from supermarkets and restaurants almost anytime of day or night. Nutritional problems tend to be due to over- rather than under-eating and life expectancy has soared to over 75 years.

However, new problems are emerging and driving changes in food policy on a global scale. The growing world population, climate change, loss of biodiversity through species extinction, food and health inequalities are but a few examples of the sorts of issues that need to be tackled. Our over-consumption of resources such as water and oil and mismanagement of land and the oceans is exceeding the capacity of the Earth's ecosystem to recover naturally. In recognition of this, there is much more interest now in scrutinizing and reducing the burden on water, land and energy resources to create more sustainable production systems. There is a need for change in the way in which we produce, distribute and consume food.

Water use is an example of the type of problem that needs to be tackled. The amount of water needed to produce certain foods, known as the **water footprint**, can be staggering. As shown in Fig. 11.1, one 250-mL glass of beer has a water footprint of 75 L. The bulk of this water is used to cultivate barley, one of the key ingredients in beer brewing. Figure 11.1 shows global averages but water footprints for the same foods can vary from one country to another. The figure also shows that it takes 15 500 L of water to produce 1 kg of beef, nearly four times as much as is needed for a kilogramme of chicken meat. All food products involving farm

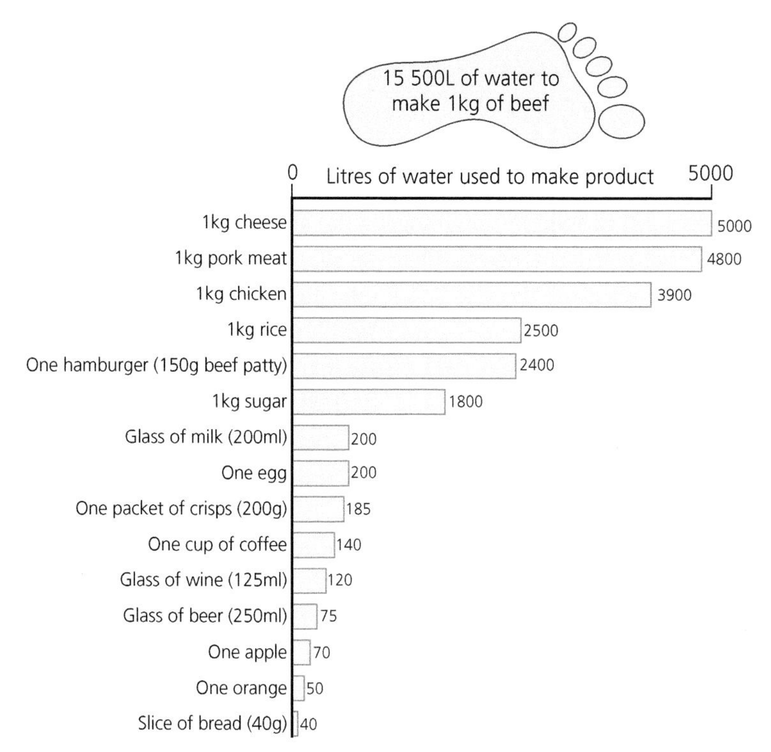

Figure 11.1 Average global water footprints for selected foods and beverages. Data from: http://www.waterfootprint.org

animals, especially cattle, require massive amounts of water in their production. Although new technologies for using water more economically are being researched, their development is outpaced by the inexorable rise in meat consumption around the world, especially in rapidly developing countries such as China and India.

The concept of food miles has proved popular with the public as a means of assessing the sustainability of food products. However, the relationship between carbon emissions from transport and food miles may not be a simple one. The mode of transport is as important as the distance. For example, sourcing fresh produce from a Mediterranean country by road for sale in the UK may lead to higher emissions than obtaining the same produce from South Africa by air.

Reducing the amount of food lost or wasted during production is another aspect that needs attention. According to the Food and Agriculture Organization of the United Nations (FAO) about one third of the foods produced globally (or 1.3 billion tonnes) is lost every year. Industrialized and developing countries waste roughly the same amount of food but for different reasons. In the developing world, food is lost during production primarily because of poor infrastructure and low levels of technology in the production systems. In the developed world, food that is otherwise safe and nutritious is wasted mainly by retailers and consumers due to quality standards that emphasize appearance and over-purchasing. In the UK, organizations such as the Waste and Resources Action Programme (WRAP) are developing new solutions to the food waste problem (for weblink, see end of chapter).

In Chapter 4 we examined some of the demographic and socio-economic factors that influence food production and food safety, such as the growth of megacities, an ageing population, increased mobility and changing life styles. A key factor in the overall picture is population growth. The world's human population of 7 billion in 2011 is predicted to climb to 10 billion by the end of the century. People will come to rely increasingly on intensive agriculture to supply enough food. In turn, the increasing numbers of animals kept for food will place even more pressure on ecosystems. Uninvited guests such as pests will add to the burden. For example, it is estimated that there are 96 million rats living in the sewers of New York City (12 for every citizen). Inevitably, food production, water and sanitation systems will be strained.

Perhaps less predictably, expansion of the population into areas previously inhabited by wildlife will create new opportunities for infectious diseases to cross over from animals into humans and spread rapidly. There are many historical examples of bacteria and viruses crossing the species barrier, of which HIV/AIDS is a good example. The HIV virus is thought to have 'jumped' species from African monkeys and chimpanzees to humans in the 1950s. The consequences have been devastating with millions of people killed by the HIV/AIDS pandemic, particularly in sub-Saharan Africa. Climate change will add to these problems by making the spread of infectious diseases more unpredictable. We can expect new infectious diseases, including foodborne illnesses, to emerge in the future.

Food inequalities

In the developed world, we concentrate on food quality and safety but much of the rest of the world worries about food security (Figs 11.2 and 11.3). Food security exists when all people, at all times, have physical, social and economic access to sufficient, safe and nutritious food (FAO).

Statistics from FAO show that the proportion of undernourished people in developing countries has halved from 33 per cent to 16 per cent in the period between 1970 and 2010. But due to population growth, the actual numbers have increased from 870 million to around 1 billion in the same 40-year period. Furthermore, the global picture masks huge regional differences. For example, more than 35 per cent of people living in sub-Saharan Africa have inadequate access to food. FAO has identified 22 countries around the world that are in protracted crisis, meaning that their people face chronic hunger due to a combination of natural disasters, war and weak governance. One of these countries is the Democratic Republic of Congo where the proportion of undernourished

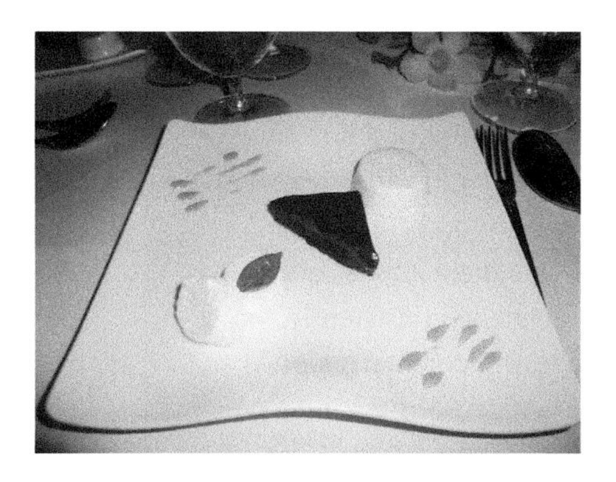

Figure 11.2 Dessert in a fine dining restaurant in a developed country.

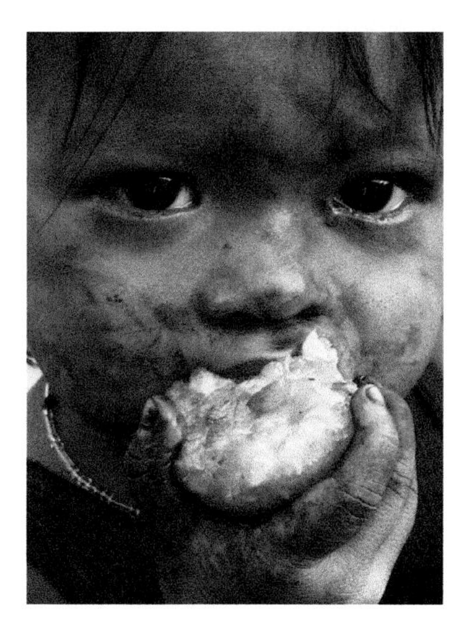

Figure 11.3 Cambodian girl eating on a municipal waste dump in Phnom Penh, 2006. Image credit: Rebecca Horn©.

people is a shocking 70 per cent (for weblink to the FAO Interactive Hunger Map of the World, see end of chapter).

By contrast, less than 5 per cent of people in North America and Europe lack sufficient food but the number of overweight and obese people is currently around 1 billion. This, too, represents a public health challenge.

Translating evidence into action: the problem of implementation

Food safety is not just about the food we eat – it is also about people and their behaviour. People working in governments, manufacturing companies and foodservice as well as the consumer all influence food safety.

As we've seen in this book, much is known about food poisoning and how to prevent it. The scientific evidence is clear and has been followed up by provision of training and guidance on safe food-handling practices. And yet, the numbers of cases of foodborne disease occurring every year are far too high and some pathogens are actually on the rise. The challenge is to change food handlers' ingrained behaviour. Many food handlers know how to wash their hands and know why it is necessary but they still don't practice hand hygiene consistently. Research undertaken in the healthcare sector has shown that implementation of good hand-hygiene practices is more likely to succeed in organizations where a safety culture is shared by all staff. Achieving such an ethos can be difficult in some businesses. Food safety is everyone's business. All members of staff in a food business share the responsibility for food safety. The long-standing anecdotal observation that many food handlers abdicate responsibility for preventing food poisoning to their supervisor or manager is simply unacceptable. Complacency and denial must be challenged.

It has been suggested that food handling should be treated like driving a car. All food handlers and food-business owners could be trained and then subjected to a stringent practical and theoretical knowledge-based test. Those who pass the test would be issued with a time-limited licence to handle food. Licence renewal would depend on evidence demonstrating that continuous professional development and updating in food-safety principles had taken place. A licensing scheme would undoubtedly be very costly and would not eliminate food poisoning entirely but it would help to reduce the burden of disease.

Conclusion

Food safety cannot be assured by a single magic bullet. Science and technology can certainly help but they cannot do so alone. Just like building a new orbital road won't solve the problem of traffic congestion in a big city, so science alone cannot provide all the answers to food-safety assurance. Socio-economic, behavioural and political factors all have a role to play. The connections between food security, safety, diet, agriculture, public health and the environment are complex. All of these have a profound influence on the safety and quality of the food we eat. Like fusion cuisine, in which flavours and ingredients from around the world are combined to create a harmonious meal, it will take a combination of approaches to solve the problems of food safety.

Weblinks

For world population projections, visit:

http://www. un. org/esa/population/unpop. htm

For water footprints, visit:
http://www. waterfootprint. org

FAO (2010). *The state of food insecurity in the world.* Available in English, French, Spanish, Russian, Arabic and Chinese from:
http://www. fao. org/publications/sofi/en
http://www. fao. org/hunger/en/

FAO (2011). *Global food losses and food waste.*
Available from:
http://www. fao. org/news/story/en/item/74192/icode/
and
http://www. fao. org/ag/ags/ags-division/publications/publication/en/?dyna_fef[uid]=74045

The Waste and Resources Action Programme (WRAP) is at:
http:www. wrap. org. uk

FSA (2010). *Food and climate change: A review of the effects of climate change on food within the remit of the Food Standards Agency.*
Available from:
http://www. food. gov. uk/science/research/supportingresearch/strategicevidenceprogramme/strategicevidenceprogramme/x02projlist/x02001/

Abbreviations and Symbols

°C degrees Celsius

°F degrees Fahrenheit

a_w water activity

cfu/ml colony forming units per millilitre or number of microbes per volume of liquid

cfu/g colony forming units per gram or number of microbes per gram of food or soil

g gram

kg kilogramme
equivalent to 1000 grams

ml millilitre

L litre
equivalent to 1000 millilitres

m metre
equivalent to 1000 millimetres

mm millimetre
equivalent to one thousandth of a metre or 1000 micrometres

μm micrometre
equivalent to one millionth of a metre or one thousandth of a millimetre

nm nanometre
equivalent to one thousandth of a micrometre

ATP adenosine triphosphate

CAP controlled atmosphere packaging

CCP Critical Control Point

CDC Centers for Disease Control and Prevention (USA)

DNA deoxyribonucleic acid

ECDC European Centre for Disease Prevention and Control

FDA Food and Drug Administration (USA)

FSA Food Standards Agency (UK)

HACCP Hazard Analysis Critical Control Point
MAP modified atmosphere packaging
RNA ribonucleic acid
VP vacuum packaging
WHO World Health Organization

Temperature conversion table (°C and °F)

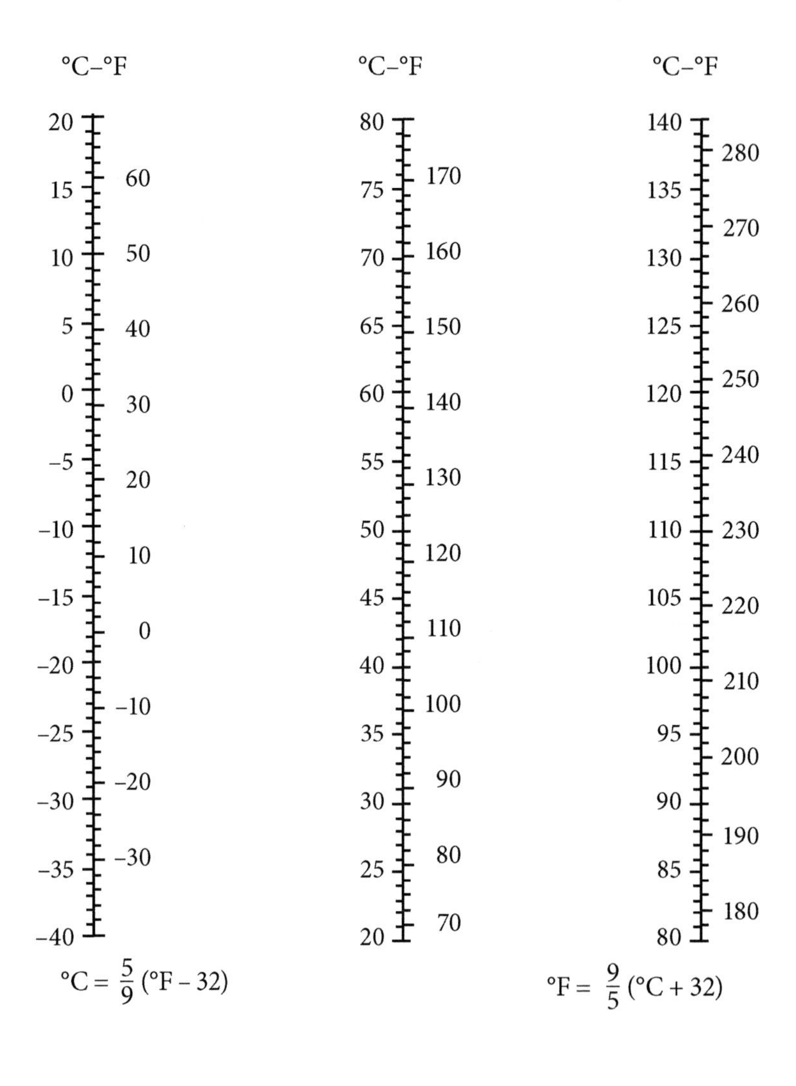

Glossary

Aerobic	In the presence of oxygen or air
Agar	An extract from seaweed made of carbohydrate and used to solidify liquid media for growing microbes in the laboratory; also used in some recipes for humans
Alga/algae	Large group of organisms ranging from the microscopic to the macroscopic, the latter often referred to as seaweed; able to make energy from sunlight by the process of photosynthesis
Amino acid	Simple organic compounds containing nitrogen that are the basic building blocks of proteins
Amino sugar	A sugar that has an amino group containing nitrogen attached to it
Anaerobic	In the absence of oxygen or air
Antibody	A highly specific molecule (usually a protein) produced in human and animal blood when a foreign substance or infectious agent enters the body
Antigen	A chemical part of a microbe or toxin that triggers the production of an antibody in human or animal blood
ATP	Adenosine triphosphate, the chemical form of energy in all living cells
a_w	See 'water activity'
Bacillus/bacilli	Rod-shaped bacterium/bacteria; there is also a genus called *Bacillus* with several food pathogens within it, such as *Bacillus cereus*
Bacteria/bacterium	Microbes that lack some of the sophisticated internal structures found in animal and plant cells
Best before date	Measure of food quality indicating shelf life and used for many dried, canned and frozen foods
Binary fission	Bacterial method of reproduction consisting of splitting the cell down the middle into two separate cells
Biofilm	Mat or community of microbes stuck together by a slimy coating

Botulinum cook	Heat treatment applied to tins of food and designed to ensure the total destruction of spores produced by *Clostridium botulinum*
Bright-field microscope	A type of light microscope that forms a dark image against a light (or bright) background
Budding	Method of reproduction usually found in yeast where a small bud forms, grows and then breaks off from the original cell
CAP or Controlled Atmosphere Packing	A method of long-term storage of fruit by modifying the gas mixture in a bulk-storage tank
Capsule	Gel-like protective coating surrounding many bacteria
Carbohydrate	Chemical compounds containing carbon, hydrogen and oxygen and found in living tissues and foods
Cardinal temperatures	The temperature growth range that characterizes each microbial species; includes the minimum, maximum and optimal temperatures for growth
Carrier	A person or animal who harbours (carries) a disease-causing organism and infects others without showing any outward symptoms of illness
Case of foodborne illness	A microorganism is isolated from a person with symptoms of a specific illness
Cell	Compartment containing a sophisticated mix of chemicals that allow it to reproduce as a unit; all plants, animals and microbes (except viruses) consist of cells
Cell membrane	Thin flexible membrane that separates cell interior from the external environment
Cell wall	Rigid outer wall of microbes separating and protecting the cell and its membrane from the environment
cfu/mL	Colony-forming units per millilitre or number of microbes per volume of liquid
cful/g	Colony-forming units per gram or number of microbes per gram of food or soil
Chromosome	String of genes, or genetic material, containing the recipe for life
Coccus/cocci	A bacterium with a spherical shape
Colon	Large intestine

Colony	Several million microbes, all piled up in a 'heap' that is visible to the naked eye
Conidia	Fungal or mould spores akin to the seeds of a plant
Conidiophores	Fungal or mould-fruiting bodies containing hundreds of conidia or spores
Controlled atmosphere	A method of preserving food by controlling the atmosphere surrounding a food product; includes vaccum packing (VP) and modified atmosphere packing (MAP)
Critical Control Point	A step in a food-preparation process that needs to be controlled to achieve safety; central to the concept of HACCP systems
Cytoplasm	Jelly-like interior of cells containing proteins, lipids, carbohydrates and minerals suspended in water
Death phase	After a microbial population has reached maximum numbers and has been in stationary phase for a while, numbers gradually start to decline
Deoxyribonucleic acid	See 'DNA'
Detergent	Surface-active chemical used for cleaning and removing grease and microbes from utensils, surfaces and equipment
Differential dye	Staining material added to microbial specimens on glass slides in order to colour bacteria differently
Dinoflagellate	Microscopic algae producing toxins that can accumulate in oysters and mussels and can lead to paralytic shellfish poisoning
Disinfectant	Powerful chemical that kills microbes
DNA	Deoxyribonucleic acid or string of nucleic acids that contain the genetic blueprint or code for life
Due diligence	Main defence used in a court of law to prove that a business has taken all reasonable precautions to avoid committing a food-safety offence
Electron microscope	A microscope that uses electron beams instead of light to magnify objects up to 100 000 times and visualize structures as close together as 1 nm
Emerging pathogen	A disease-causing microbe that was not known historically but has emerged recently to cause illness

Endospore	Heat-resistant structures found inside some bacteria
Enterotoxin	Toxins or poisons that affect the gut
Eukaryote	Organism that has specialized organelles or miniature organs within the cell; includes animals, plants, fungi and protozoa
Faecal–oral route of transmission	Spread of microbes from faeces to the mouth, often via human hands
Fimbria/fimbriae	Fringe-like protrusions that help bacteria to attach to surfaces and gut cells
Fitness to work	A person's capacity to work without risk to their own or others' health
Flagella/flagellae	Long, whip-like tails that help bacteria to move or swim through liquids
Fungus/fungi	A group of microbes that includes yeasts, moulds and mushrooms
Gastroenteritis	Most common symptoms of food poisoning, including diarrhoea, abdominal cramps, vomiting and sometimes fever
Gene	A unit of hereditary material inside every microbial, animal, plant and human cell
Genome	All the genes contained within a microbe, plant or animal
Germinate	When conditions are favourable, the spores of some bacteria germinate to form vegetative cells and multiply
Growth media	Liquid and semi-solid 'soups' used to grow microbes in the laboratory
Guideline	Advice concerning the microbiological acceptability of a food; issued by government agencies and professional bodies to encourage best practice
HACCP system	Hazard Analysis Critical Control Point system of assuring food safety by predicting what could go wrong and how to prevent it
Hazard	A source of danger. Hazards in foods can be physical (e.g. a piece of glass), chemical (e.g. pesticide residues) or biological (e.g. *Salmonella* sp.)
Hypha/hyphae	Branched, thread-like, tubular filaments produced by moulds

Immunoassay	A method of detecting microbes based on antibodies
Improvement Notice	Written warning issued by an Environmental Health Practitioner (food inspector) to a business that is not complying with food law
Indicator organisms	Harmless microbes that are easy to detect and are used as surrogates for estimating the quality of food or the likelihood of pathogen presence
Infection	An illness caused by multiplication of microbes in the body
Infective dose	Minimum number of microbes needed to cause symptoms of illness
Intoxication	Illness caused by a microbial toxin produced in a food or in the gut
Lag phase	A 'warm up' period when microbes prepare for reproduction and multiplication; precedes the log phase
Log phase	The most rapid phase of microbial growth when numbers increase exponentially (or logarithmically)
Mesophiles	Microbes that grow most rapidly at moderate temperatures, usually between 28°C and 43°C
Microbe	A tiny living thing, usually invisible to the naked eye (from the Greek *micro*, small, and *bios*, life)
Microbiologist	A person excited about very tiny living things
Microbiology	The study of microscopic forms of life, including bacteria, fungi, viruses, protozoa and some algae. Ideal career choice for people with obsessive–compulsive tendencies
Microflora	Mix of microbes typically found in a habitat or specified environment (e.g. in the human gut)
Modified atmosphere packaging (MAP)	A method of food preservation based on modifying the gas composition in the food package; carbon dioxide in the gas mixture slows down microbial growth
Mother cell	Bacterial cells that form hardy spores inside them
Mould	A type of fungus often growing in filaments
Mycelium	A mass of hyphae or microscopic filaments produced by moulds

Neurotoxin	Toxin or poison that affects the nervous system
Non-proteolytic	An organism unable to break down proteins readily; usually refers to strains of *Clostridium botulinum* that can grow at chill temperatures
Optimum temperature	The ideal temperature for a microbe to multiply rapidly
Outbreak	Two or more related cases of illness
Pathogen	A microbe that causes illness in plants, animals or humans
Peptidoglycan	Complex organic compound consisting of amino acids and sugars and responsible for conferring rigidity to bacterial cell walls
Pilus/pili	Hair-like protrusions that help bacteria to stick to surfaces and other cells
Plasmid	DNA-containing hereditary material present in some bacteria in addition to the main genome contained within the chromosomes
Polysaccharide	A type of carbohydrate that consists of long chains of monosaccharide or sugar units
Prebiotic	Ingredients that stimulate the growth of beneficial bacteria in the gut
Probiotic	Live microbes, usually lactic acid bacteria, reported to be beneficial for gut health
Prohibition Notice	Order issued by an Environmental Health Practitioner (food inspector) for a business to close down part or all of its operations due to severe breaches in food-safety law
Prokaryote	Organism that has no specialized compartments within the cell; cell contents free-float in the cytoplasm; includes all bacteria
Protein	Class of organic compounds consisting of long chains of amino acids. Important in cell structure and human nutrition
Proteolytic	Able to degrade (break down) proteins; opposite of non-proteolytic
Protozoa	Microbes with sexual life cycles that are more complex than those of bacteria or fungi; many form resistant cysts that help the organism to survive
Quorum sensing	A primitive form of communication between bacteria using small signalling molecules

Resolution	Resolving power or ability of a microscope to detect two objects that are close together as separate objects
Resolving power	Ability of a microscope to detect two objects that are close together as separate objects
Ribonucleic acid	See 'RNA'
Ribosome	Structures within a cell responsible for making proteins, using DNA as blueprints
Risk	An estimate of the likely occurrence of a hazard or danger
RNA	Ribonucleic acid; plays a role in translating DNA into proteins via the ribosomes; acts as genetic material in some viruses
Selective media	Growth media containing chemicals that allow some microbes to multiply but stop others from growing
Serotype	A subgroup of bacteria within a species with specific chemical structures on the cell surface that allow classification using antibodies
Severity (of hazard)	Used to describe the level of danger presented by a hazard
Shelf life	The period of time during which a food is microbiologically safe and retains its sensory properties (flavour, texture, aroma) under specified storage conditions
Specification	Microbiological condition of a food specified by a buyer or user of food
Sporadic case	A sick person that has no known connection with another person infected by the same microbe
Spore	Seed-like structures produced by moulds and some bacteria that enable the microbes to survive harsh environmental conditions; bacterial spores are more heat resistant than fungal spores
Sputum	Mucus or pus coughed up from the lungs of a (usually infected) patient
Standard	Microbiological condition of a food specified by law and enforced by regulatory agencies
Stationary phase	After rapid growth during the log phase, a microbial population stops multiplying and is in stationary phase when cells are still metabolically active but do not reproduce

Sterilization	Complete removal or destruction of all microbes present in a food or clinical specimen
Streaking out	A laboratory technique used to separate and purify microorganisms from mixed cultures (see Fig. 3.2)
Super-spreader	A person or animal that spreads disease-causing organisms to others without showing any outward symptoms of illness; also referred to as super-shedder
Temperature danger zone	Temperature zone between 5°C and 63°C deemed dangerous because it allows microbes to multiply rapidly; the longer a food is allowed to remain in this temperature zone, the more likely it is that microbial growth will occur
Toxin	Poison
Use-by date	Measure of food safety used for many perishable foods
Vacuum packaging (VP)	A method of food preservation by extracting all of the air from a food package
Vegetative cells	Heat-sensitive cells that are capable of rapid multiplication; spores form inside vegetative cells
Virion	Virus (see below)
Virulence	Ability of a microrganism to cause disease
Virus	A parasitic infectious agent, several times smaller than bacteria, that hijacks the cell's machinery to reproduce itself; viruses can attack plants, animals and bacteria
Water activity (a_w)	The amount of water available for a microbe to grow (not the same as water content)
Water footprint	Amount of water needed to produce a product
Yeast	A single-celled, oval-shaped fungus that divides by budding or fission; wine and beer would not exist without it

Appendix: exercise and quiz answers

Exercise answers for Chapter 1

The differences between home cooking, catering and food manufacturing

Differences in:	Home cooking	Catering	Food manufacturing
Scale	Small scale: e.g. cooking for a family of 3–6 people	Medium scale: e.g. 70 covers in a fine-dining restaurant or 200 guests at a wedding	Large scale: e.g. thousands of portions of ready meals, distributed nationally and internationally
Timing	Meals often eaten as soon as cooked. Leftovers may be kept for a few days. Family gatherings and holidays may necessitate some preparation in advance	Fine dining: individual portions prepared for immediate consumption. Larger events: preparation 1–5 days in advance is common	Foods often prepared with a minimum shelf life of 1–2 weeks, sometimes several years (as in canning)
Location	Prepared and eaten on the same premises	May be eaten on the premises or transported for short distances nationally	Foods not eaten on premises. Often transported and distributed internationally
Accountability when things go wrong	None, except moral responsibility to family and friends	The Food Safety Act in the UK. Similar laws in many developed countries	The Food Safety Act in the UK. Similar laws in many developed countries
Possible consequences	Illness and possibly death of family and friends	Illness and death of many customers, fines, loss of reputation, loss of business, jail	Illness and death of many customers, large fines, loss of reputation, drop in sales, bankruptcy, business closure, jail, death penalty in some countries

Quiz answers for Chapter 2

1. What different types of microbes are there? Name as many groups as you can think of.

   A: Bacteria, yeasts, moulds, protozoa, algae, viruses.

2. What are the differences between bacteria, yeasts and moulds? (Tip: Comment on the differences in shape, size and internal structures.)

   A: Shapes: Bacteria can be spherical (cocci), rod-shaped (bacilli), comma-shaped (vibrio) or spirillar (corkscrew-shaped). Yeasts are ovoid. Moulds

consist of branched filaments (hyphae), often forming a mycelium. Of the three groups of microbes, bacteria are smallest and the moulds are biggest with the yeasts in-between. A microscope is needed to see them all. Bacteria and moulds form spores. Yeasts and moulds are eukaryotic and bacteria are prokaryotic. Prokaryotes have cell walls, cell membranes, cytoplasm, DNA in a chromosome and ribosomes. Eukaryotes are more complex and have a nucleus as well as many other specialized organelles.

3. Can you use a standard light microscope to see 'flu' viruses? Explain your answer.

   A: **No. Viruses are too small to be seen under the standard light microscope.**

4. Why is it important to know whether bacteria are Gram negative or Gram positive?

   A: **Gram-staining is the first step in the identification of a bacterium.**

5. Are microbial cells visible under a standard light microscope?

   A: **Yes but they are often transparent and colourless, so dyes are used to improve contrast.**

Quiz answers for Chapter 3

1. Where can we find microbes?

   A: **Microbes are all around us, in the air we breathe, the water we drink and the food we eat. They are on inert surfaces and on and in our bodies.**

2. What conditions do you think would encourage the growth of microbes?

   A: **Water, warmth, nutrients (food).**

3. If you exposed nutrient agar plates and malt extract agar plates to air, would you expect to see differences between them after incubation? If so, why?

   A: **Yes. Nutrient agar is a general-purpose medium and will support growth of bacteria, yeasts and moulds. Malt extract agar is acidic and so will support growth of moulds, which are more acid tolerant than bacteria.**

4. Name five examples of inert surfaces on everyday objects that may have microbes on them.

   A: **Any five from:**
   - **grab rails on trains and buses;**
   - **handbags and rucksacks;**
   - **handles (on doors, cupboards, lockers, windows, shopping baskets);**
   - **keypads and touchscreens for cash and ticket machines;**

- electrical switches (for lights, fans, radiators);
- lift (elevator) buttons;
- remote controls for TVs and other electrical equipment;
- pens;
- telephones;
- money (coins and notes);
- sink taps (kitchen and bathroom);
- sinks (kitchen and bathroom);
- soap dispensers.

Examples from kitchens would also be correct, for example:

- touchpads/controls for appliances (e.g. microwave and conventional ovens);
- all handles (fridges, cupboards, doors);
- cleaning sponges, cloths and brushes (especially when damp);
- dishcloths and towels (especially when damp);
- floor mops;
- staff clothing, uniforms, aprons;
- chopping boards made from all materials including wood and plastics;
- mixing bowls (glass, ceramic, plastic);
- utensils, all tools with handles (e.g. knives);
- delicatessen slicers;
- work surfaces made of granite, marble and stainless steel;
- waste bins;
- papers and charts (recipes, cookbooks, food orders);
- any sites where dust is allowed to settle.

5. Name a disease-causing microbe that can live on human skin and cause food poisoning.

   A: ***Staphylococcus aureus*** **(should be spelt correctly).**

Quiz answers for Chapter 4

1. The number of foodborne cases of illness occurring globally is unacceptably high. Name five possible reasons for this.

   A. **Any five from the following list would be correct: improved surveillance, global population growth, intensive farming, increasing urbanization, increasing numbers of vulnerable people, increased mobility of people and foods, emerging pathogens, changing lifestyles, misbehaviour by food handlers.**

2. Name five groups of people who are more likely to get sick and whose illness is likely to be more severe than in a healthy adult male.

   A. Any five from the following list would be correct:
   - **the elderly or anyone over the age of 60 years;**
   - **young children and babies;**
   - **pregnant women and their unborn children;**
   - **people with immune systems suppressed by medication or illness (e.g. cancer patients, HIV-positive individuals, diabetics, transplant patients)**
   - **people on antacid medication;**
   - **alcoholics and drug abusers;**
   - **the malnourished (e.g. the sick, the homeless, people in long-term residential care)**
   - **the undernourished (mainly in developing countries).**

3. Which four foodborne microbes are most often responsible for causing disease?

   A. *Salmonella, Campylobacter, Escherichia coli* and *Listeria*

4. Name three food groups most often responsible for outbreaks of foodborne disease.

   A. Any combination of the following would be correct: poultry (chicken, turkey, duck, other poultry), red meats (lamb, beef, pork), complex foods, fish and shellfish, milk, eggs.

5. Food safety is a shared responsibility. Name the three main factors that must be in place to underpin food safety for all.

   A. Government, consumers, food industry/foodservice.

Quiz answers for Chapter 5

1. Name the two bacteria and the single food source most often responsible for food poisoning worldwide.

   A: *Campylobacter, Salmonella*. Raw chicken.

2. Outbreaks of foodborne illness are often caused by more than one cause. Name the two factors most often associated with *Salmonella* poisoning.

   A: Undercooking and cross-contamination.

3. What is the preferred method of washing up after preparing raw chicken and why?

   A: A dishwasher is better than washing up by hand because of the higher temperatures achieved in a machine. *Salmonella* can survive in hand-hot water for a long time.

4. Which pair of foods must always be kept separate to avoid cross-contamination? (Select one pair only)
   - Raw potatoes and raw stewing steak.
   - Cooked chicken and a dressed, mixed-leaf salad.
   - Raw chicken portions and fresh tomato salad.
   - Raw, washed spring onions and cooked roast beef.

   A: **Raw chicken portions and fresh tomato salad.**

5. Which of the following foods served at a buffet is most likely to cause food poisoning? (Select one only)
   - Tuna and sweetcorn salad made with bottled mayonnaise.
   - French bread.
   - Mixed green salad dressed with oil and vinegar.
   - Barbequed chicken wings.
   - Crisps and peanuts.

   A: **Barbequed chicken wings.**

Exercise answers for Chapter 6: The humble sandwich

Exercise 1: Sandwiches and their fillings

Sandwich	Potential hazards	Alternative filling
Bagel filled with cold-smoked salmon, cream cheese and watercress	*Listeria* grows at fridge temperatures and has been isolated from cold-smoked salmon and unpasteurized cheese; watercress may be contaminated with enteric (gut) bacteria such as VTEC	Hot-smoked or canned salmon. Wash watercress thoroughly or replace with thinly sliced onion. Always use pasteurized cream cheese
Baguette with tuna, cucumber and mayonnaise with flat-leaf parsley and spring onions	Tuna is usually canned, so low risk. Cucumber, parsley and spring onions may be contaminated with enteric bacteria such as VTEC. If unpasteurized, mayonnaise may contain *Salmonella*	Wash fresh produce thoroughly, peel cucumber and/or replace with fermented vegetables such as gherkins, capers or olives. Always use bottled (pasteurized) mayonnaise
Club sandwich made with toasted white bread, smoked ham, sliced cheddar, mayonnaise and lettuce	Ham may be contaminated with *Listeria*, especially if cold-smoked or low in salt. Likewise for cheese, if made with unpasteurized milk. Lettuce may be contaminated with enterics, including VTEC and *Salmonella*	Hot-smoked or canned ham and cheese made from pasteurized milk. Wash lettuce thoroughly or replace with Branston pickle or gherkins. Always use bottled (pasteurized) mayonnaise

Egg and cress with mayonnaise on brown bread	Cress may be contaminated with VTEC	Egg should be thoroughly cooked until both the white and yolk are hard. Replace cress with thoroughly washed lettuce or fermented vegetables
Falafel, hummus and coriander in pita bread	Possible enterics (VTEC, *Salmonella*) in hummus and coriander	Use pasteurized hummus and thoroughly wash coriander or replace with washed and peeled cucumber
Hot wrap with Mexican chicken and jalapeño peppers	Improperly cooked chicken may contain *Salmonella* or *Campylobacter*. Jalapeño peppers may be contaminated with *Salmonella*	Ensure chicken is properly cooked, using a food thermometer (see Ch. 8). Replace fresh peppers with bottled (pasteurized) peppers
Add your own sandwich examples here:(model answers not possible here)		

Exercise 2: Should sandwiches sold in a hospital café be made by volunteers?

Risk factors associated with sandwich making	
Sandwiches made by volunteers	**Pre-packed sandwiches from commercial supplier**
• Volunteers are often untrained or poorly trained • High-quality ingredients from reputable suppliers, including 'certificates of compliance' – would volunteers know how to check for these? • Shelf-life of ingredients – would volunteers check these? • HACCP system may be unfamiliar to volunteers • Can due diligence be demonstrated in a court of law if there is an outbreak? • Customers are hospital visitors, outpatients including pregnant women and children, hospital patients who can walk. High proportion of vulnerable groups • How long are the sandwiches stored after preparation? At what temperature? Who checks this? • How is cleaning done? Etc.	If enforcement officers find problems with premises, business can be closed down Prosecution in cases of outbreaks Fines, imprisonment

Taking all of the above risk factors into consideration, which of the two methods of making sandwiches would you select for the hospital café?

A: Pre-packed sandwiches from commercial supplier – too many risks associated with volunteers.

Exercise 3: Complying with the law

1. Would knowledge of the law change your decision made in Exercise 2?

   A: **No, decision should be the same. Food safety is a shared responsibility.**

2. Do you think that this law helps to prevent *Listeria* outbreaks?

   A: **Yes if inspection regimes are implemented and breaches of the law prosecuted.**

   - **Discuss your answers with other students on your course.**

No model answer.

Exercise model answer for Chapter 7

A: **Send the chef home and tell him not to return to work less than 48 hours after the last symptoms of illness. Call the cleaner or another member of staff not involved in food handling, if possible, and ask them to clean the washroom thoroughly including the use of a chlorine-based disinfectant. Inform all staff of the incident and enquire if gastrointestinal symptoms have been experienced by others. Any staff with symptoms should be sent home and instructed not to return to work within 48 hours of the last symptom. All remaining staff should be instructed to be extra vigilant about hand hygiene. Record complaints of gastrointestinal illness from customers and, if these increase, notify public health authorities and get help from a food-safety advisor.**

Quiz answers for Chapter 7

1. Which of the following is most likely to cause food poisoning?

   A: **c. A platter of fresh seafood, including raw oysters.**

2. If food is contaminated with food-poisoning bacteria, you can normally tell by:

   A: **d. None of the above.**

3. *Staphylococcus aureus* bacteria are most likely to cause food poisoning when present in which food/beverage?

   A: **b. A cream cake left overnight at room temperature.**

4. Name three groups of food-poisoning bacteria that are easily controlled (killed) by heat.

   A: **Many possible answers, for example *Salmonella*, *Campylobacter*, verocytotoxin-producing *Escherichia coli* (VTEC), norovirus, etc.**

5. You've been served a thoroughly cooked chicken from a farm recently infected with 'bird flu'. Would you eat it? Explain your answer.

   A: Yes. There is no evidence that bird flu is foodborne. The virus is transmitted through respiratory means.

Quiz answers for Chapter 8

1. A chef is seen smoking on the pavement in front of a restaurant. He is wearing protective overalls, an apron and blue plastic gloves. What is wrong with this and why?

   A: There are several problems with the chef's behaviour:
   - **Kitchen uniforms and aprons should not be worn outside the kitchens where they could pick up dust and dirt that would then be transferred to food and the kitchen environment.**
   - **Plastic gloves are intended to protect food from contamination by microbes on the food handler's hands. If the food handler smokes with the gloves on, microbes from his mouth will be transferred to the gloves and then to food when he returns to work. Equally, the gloves protect the food handler from contaminating his hands during preparation of high-risk foods. By keeping the gloves on, he risks infecting himself. Therefore, smoking with the gloves on defeats the point of wearing them in the first place.**

Exercise model answers for Chapter 8

Exercise 1

Microbial control measures	
Milk and milk products	
Pasteurized milk	Heating to pasteurization temperatures (e.g. 72°C for 15 seconds) Chill storage below 5°C
UHT milk	Heating to 135°C for 2 seconds Aseptic packaging
Sweetened condensed milk in a can	Evaporation and addition of sugar to reduce water activity Heating in a sealed can (e.g. 115°C for 30 minutes) Anaerobic atmosphere
Dried milk powder	Heating during evaporation Drying to a water activity below which most microbes don't grow

Cream	Heating to pasteurization temperatures (e.g. 72°C for 15 seconds) Separation of fat from whey (aqueous fraction)
Yogurt	Heating to pasteurization temperatures (e.g. 72°C for 15 seconds) Acidification by lactic acid bacteria in the starter culture Some yogurts are pasteurized after fermentation is complete Chill storage below 5°C
Cheese	Heating to pasteurization temperatures (e.g. 72°C for 15 seconds) Starter culture produces lactic acid Salting Release of whey reduces water activity (a_w) Chill storage below 5°C
Meat and meat products	
VP fresh beef joint for catering trade	Lack of oxygen Chill storage below 5°C
MA packed fresh pork roast in retailer's pack	Carbon dioxide in gas atmosphere inhibits bacterial growth Chill storage below 5°C
Canned corned beef	Botulinum cook, i.e. heating in a sealed can (e.g. 115°C for 30 minutes)
Frozen minced beef	Freezing arrests microbial growth, water is solid
Pâté	Heating above 72°C for at least 2 minutes (usually baked for much longer than this) VP or MA packaging Chill storage below 5°C
Sweetcure bacon rashers	Nitrite and salt to preserve the meat As sweetcure is low-salt, chill storage below 5°C is necessary
Salami slices in retail pack	Fermentation with starter culture produces acid Salt and spices inhibit bacterial growth Drying reduces a_w
Fish and fish products	
Frozen, oven-ready breaded cod fillets	Freezing arrests microbial growth, water is solid
Canned tuna	Botulinum cook, i.e. heating in a sealed can (e.g. 115°C for 30 minutes)
Bacalao (dried fish)	Salt inhibits microbial growth Drying to a water activity below which most microbes don't grow
Rollmops (marinated herring)	Marinade often contains vinegar (acetic acid) Spices, herbs Chill storage below 5°C
Thai fish sauce	Fermentation by starter culture reduces pH Salt inhibits microbial growth Reduced a_w

VP, cold-smoked salmon	Phenolic compounds in cold cure Chill storage below 5°C Lack of oxygen
Sushi	Chill storage below 5°C(may have been previously frozen to reduce parasite larvae)
Wheat and wheat products: from noodles to strudels!	
Madeira cake	Heating during baking Low a_w
Sliced sourdough bread	Heating during baking Acidity produced by sourdough starter culture
Chocolate éclair	Heating of pastry during baking Chill storage below 5°C
Prawn and mayonnaise vol-au-vents	Heating of pastry during baking Chill storage below 5°C
Spaghetti	Drying to a water activity below which most microbes don't grow
Fresh tortellini filled with spinach and ricotta in MAP	Parts of filling (e.g. spinach) may have been heated Carbon dioxide in gas atmosphere inhibits bacterial growth Chill storage below 5°C
Wheat flour	Dried product at a water activity below which most microbes don't grow

Exercise 2

1. Question A: Which ingredients in the mousse are high risk in terms of food safety and what was the most likely source of the *Salmonella*? Explain your answer.
2. Question B: Was the cool larder adequate for storing mousse? Explain your answer.
3. Question C: What recommendations would you make to your line manager regarding the preparation and storage of the mousses for the gala dinner? Could some of the ingredients be replaced with safer alternatives?

Answer A: **Sugar and couverture are low risk as they are dry and/or low in water activity. The higher risk ingredients are egg, cream and milk. The cream and milk have been pasteurized, so provided they have been stored at temperatures below 5°C and are within their 'use by' dates, they should be medium risk. The highest risk comes from fresh eggs, which may harbour *Salmonella*.**

Answer B: **No. The larder was not cool enough to inhibit growth of bacteria even in those mousses that did not contain *Salmonella*. Numbers of bacteria in the larder-stored mousse were nearly 10 times higher than in freshly**

prepared mousses. In mousses prepared without heating, numbers rose more than 10 times between the day of preparation and overnight storage in the larder and *Salmonella* was present throughout.

Answer C: **If fresh eggs are to be used, the preferred method of making the mousse must include a heating step. Additional reassurance could be achieved by using Lion Code Quality eggs but this is no cast-iron guarantee that the eggs will be *Salmonella*-free. Alternatively, pasteurized egg products could be used. Arrangements must be made for adequate chilling. If this is not possible, an alternative dessert that does not require chilling should be developed. Additional precautions could include specifying and checking of temperatures and 'use by' dates on pasteurized products on delivery and rejecting all deliveries that do not comply with specifications.**

Exercise 3

There is no model answer for this exercise as a multitude of correct answers are possible.

Index

Indexer: Dr Laurence Errington

Note: page references in italics are to the glossary.